Ruptured Cerebral ANEURYSM:
Fire in the Brain

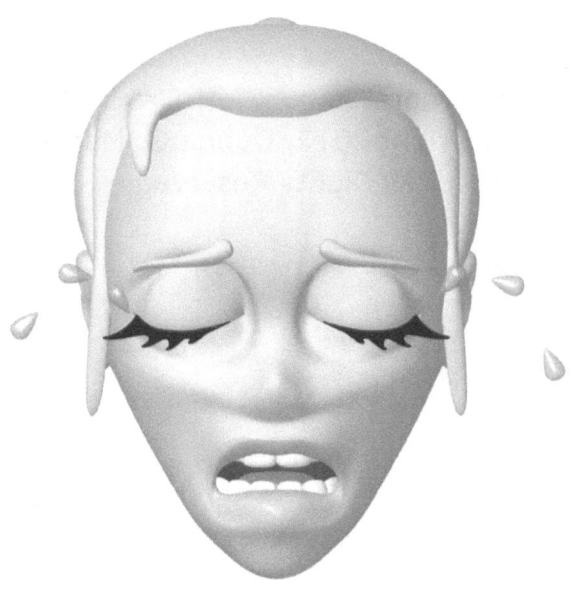

A true story by

Donna G. Magee

Attempts were made to contact everyone of professional prominence included in this story. It was not possible, so out of fairness and the need to be consistent, all professional names and locations were changed, in the interest of anonymity.

ISBN 978-1-300-33341-8

9 781300 333418

Ruptured Brain Aneurysm:

Fire in the Brain

The Attack & the Aftermath

This is a true story recounting the first four or five years following my brain incident; from the lightning fast onset of my ruptured brain aneurysm through craniotomy surgery and ultimately, a long and difficult physical effort to battle the numerous complications in order to survive.

In loving gratitude to my husband, my family and Marine Corps League, Detachment 1128, forever a part of my life.

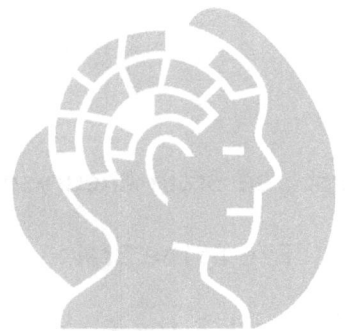

Ruptured cerebral aneurysm –

Abnormal dilated segment of a blood vessel surrounding the brain which has widened and expanded to the point of bursting, causing blood to escape into the space between the brain and the wall surrounding it resulting in a subarachnoid hemorrhage which compresses and damages the tissue of the brain.

Dedication

I dedicate this book to all brain aneurysm survivors; to all of us confronted with the sudden and violent upheaval as the "A" card slams into us, forever changing our lives.

A ruptured brain aneurysm is horrifying, striking without warning, quickly throwing us into a world of intense pain; a world where everything is familiar, but so very strange.

It attacks with the force of a cannonball fired directly into the top of our head - crushing, maiming and destroying so much of our very being.

Although the medical odds are not in our favor, as survivors, we can still flourish, as a distinct specialty group of the determined and courageous. We have been drastically dented; not totally destroyed, and grasp each remaining day of our life with remarkable inner strength and a profound sense of integrity and humanity.

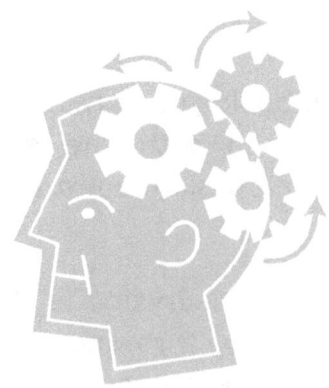

Craniotomy –

Surgical operation in which part of the skull is removed in order to access the brain.

Preface

As a survivor, I have often been told how lucky I am, to still be alive, and after spending an entire year researching this horrendous medical incident, assisted by the nation's top neurological centers and institutes, I am fortunate, indeed. I write this book in part, because survival comes with a price – a huge price. A void in what was once excitement and energetic enthusiasm remains to this day. A daily routine is impossible. The searing pain from what seemed like a lightning bolt that struck my head sends a constant reminder – I have no self sustaining directions. I must rely, in part, on someone, for things that were once as repetitive and simple as cooking and driving.

I was painfully surprised at the number of complications that would surface; unable to understand them. It was impossible to predict them. My extensive team of physicians were precise in saying they did not know what form any future damages would manifest themselves in. Survival statistics are so low that there is no guide to turn to; no professional medical curriculum, no way to predict what might, could and would happen.

After crossing my three year 'anniversary,' I decided that I had to write my story; for survivors like myself, so that they might be better prepared, enduring a litany of complications; knowing they aren't alone. Just as important in sharing my story are the family members, friends, neighbors, co-workers and care givers that have the compassionate and exasperating task of caring for, coping with, working with and living with us without benefit of knowing what each day will bring.

I journeyed through my survival in a predominately trial and error method. Only after some medical disaster presented itself did I find out that it was a latent complication from the aneurysm. In retrospect, it would have been tremendously beneficial for my family to know some of the potential complications.

I have corresponded with many survivors across the states and found that we had as many similarities as differences. We all had varying degrees of damage, but the one striking fact was that none of us knew what could happen to us down the road. We are all the same in the sense that we are physically blocked from returning to life as we knew it. We are all different in our sets and scopes of permanent damages, but we have all been blessed with that gift to still be alive, to keep trying and to never give up. We are all held back in various ways. Our lifelong personality structure has been changed, held captive by our own brain. Specific traits we possessed all our lives are now gone! Lost in the damage? Altered by the surgery? We will never know, yet we are all convinced that the 'old self' is still in there, buried deep among the packing and metal we now house in our heads.

We all have weakened immune systems, making it dangerous to catch a common cold. We can never, ever put a decongestant in our mouth again. To do so would initiate immediate and probably fatal consequences, constricting blood flow to the brain. Any future maladies of the brain would be extremely difficult to find and diagnose; an MRI is out of the realm of testing; most of us have non-compatible aneurysm clips in our brain.

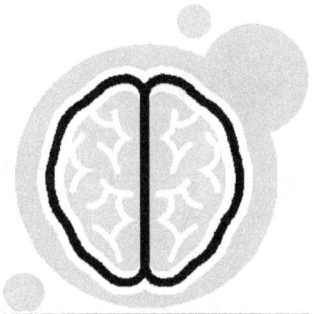

Hydrocephalus –

Abnormal and excessive accumulation of cerebrospinal fluid in the brain, in this case, resulting from a subarachnoid hemorrhage, causing extreme pain from intercranial pressure inside the skull

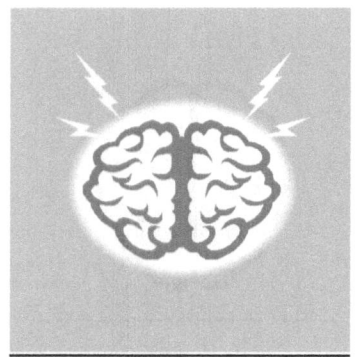

<u>Subarachnoid hemorrhage</u> –

Consequence of a ruptured cerebral aneurysm as blood from the aneurysm pulses into the area of the skull surrounding the brain and mixes with cerebrospinal fluid. The sudden build up of pressure causes loss of consciousness and/or death

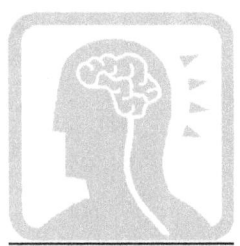

<u>Vasospasm</u> -

Abnormal constriction of the blood vessels of the brain resulting in tissue damage and destruction caused by diminished blood flow to the brain

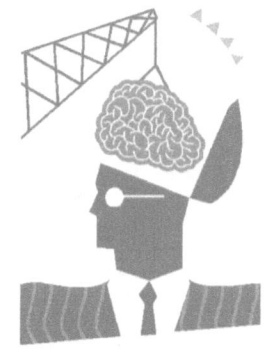

Peripheral neuropathy -

Damage to and destruction of the peripheral nervous system neurons serving the limbs and organs, in this case, as a result of a brain hemorrhage

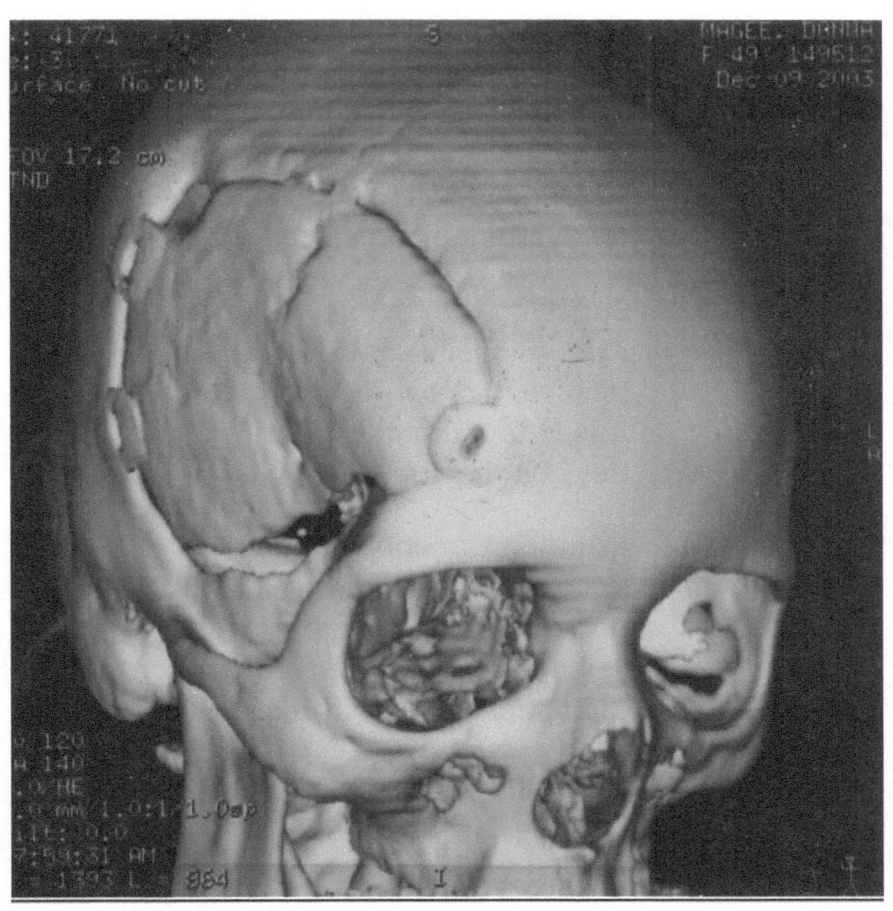

My skull, about 10 months after surgery.

Contents

Part One

The explosion inside my head
Cerebral volcano and brain surgery
Surrounded by fog
Home strange home

There was nothing unusual about the clear, crisp Saturday morning of January 25, 2003. The sun was desperately trying to peek through the stubborn layer of clouds as I made the easy ten minute drive to work. It was a routine part of my normal work schedule to meet with clients every other Saturday morning; those unable to make it into the office during the week because of their own work schedules, parenting demands or other obligations.

I pulled into the same parking space I had claimed as my own for the past three years, put my new Pontiac Vibe into park, turned off the ignition, removed the keys, grabbed purse and briefcase, gave the door a gentle push and stepped up onto the sidewalk.

I had that natural exuberance about me; that clarity of compassion and understanding that is a predominant factor in my field, the funeral arena. Having lost my own father 3 years prior, I was intimately connected to the sense of grief and loss, as well as the numerous details that death encompasses.

In the split second amount of time it would have taken to complete my third step, *my head suddenly exploded!* I was momentarily paralyzed, crippled by the lightening fast, intense, burning explosion. My eyes felt as if they were being ripped from their sockets; my ears screaming, as if someone had driven a stake into them. My eyes fogged over, as if I was looking through a thick sheet of plastic. I felt the immediate inferno as my body temperature raced well past the 98.6 mark.

My crowning glory had seemingly turned into a volcanic eruption, spewing lava with an unbelievable fusion of heat and pain. The dizziness and nausea quickly followed. After what could have been a few seconds or several minutes, I looked down to see if perhaps I'd stepped on a live wire. All I saw on the ground was the floating image of my purse and briefcase; nothing that could have caused *this!*

Little did I know that this was the exact moment in time that my life would be changed forever. The past 48 years, 7 months and 5 days would be as unfamiliar to me as the surface of Jupiter.

As was habit, I used the isolated, side entrance to the building; the section of the building that houses the administrative offices. There was no one around to reach out to, especially on a Saturday morning. So, in a series of slow motion movements, I gathered my belongings and forced myself to make it inside the building, the Seth Kersey Funeral Home. My office was on the left, just a dozen steps away. I struggled with each step and finally reached my destination, collapsing into my chair. As I sat with my elbows planted on the desk, my head propped up in my hands; I tried to hurry this episode along. Streaks of bright lights were now added to the blurry layer of film, making vision practically obscure. The weekend manager on duty came in to say hello and questioned my unnatural pale, queasy state. I tried to explain my predicament; what had happened, and he was quick to alert me to the fact that there was a new strain of the flu going around. He suggested that perhaps I should go home, take some cold and flu medicine and sleep it off.

No, I insisted, I have a family arriving any minute. *I have to do my job!* Having never had a serious illness or medical condition in my life, I was certain this was a spell of something that had a short duration, hopefully a very short duration.

Eventually I convinced myself that maybe it was the flu, it seemed likely. I didn't know. I had always managed to steer clear of it before. I was quick to realize that if it was the flu, it would eventually pass, as soon as I could get home and crawl into bed for a day or so.

Fighting through the blur, I stepped into the adjoining conference room to perform a quick survey; ensure everything was in place for my meeting. Client file packet, calculator, pens, legal pads, Kleenex and mints, all nicely arranged at one end of the massive cherry surface. The middle section neatly housed a respectable assortment of trade publications, manuals and books that showcased every funeral option available.

I adjusted the dimmer switch for the proper, respectable amount of lighting and opened the adjoining door to the beverage center. After a quick inventory of juices, I staggered back to my office to wait. And hope. Hope that this *flu* would ease up just enough so that I could make it through this consultation.

Kay and Patty would be arriving any minute and I was supposed to evaluate their mother's life insurance coverage. What company? Had they changed names, been bought out? Is the policy still in effect? Who are the named beneficiaries? What is the actual death benefit? Is there enough coverage to pay for a decent funeral? That was the leading reason for most of these meetings. Inadequate life insurance. A family's need to know - how much they would possibly have to scrape together to pay for the funeral.

My head was getting worse by the second, sending me into a frenzy of persistent pain. This just can't be happening! Being a funeral consultant doesn't allow you time to be sick. The cycle of death goes on 24 hours a day.

I've got to get through this, then I can go home and take something for this dreadful flu and lay down. As I prayed for temporary relief, my clients arrived.

These two sisters needed and deserved my utmost attention, having chosen this mortuary for their mother's service. Even though she was elderly and sick, we all hoped and prayed that death would not arrive for many more years. The major issue was the status of some very old life insurance policies, circa 1940. So many of these companies of old had since gone out of business, been sold or gone through numerous name changes. It was part of my expertise to track down the current insurer, ascertain current policy values, named beneficiaries and specific claims procedures as each company had pretty stringent regulations for filing a death claim.

Through some incredible miracle far beyond my scope of comprehension, I got through the hour long meeting, placed the policies in my office file, ensured that it was securely locked and stumbled out to my car. Had it been a weekday, I would have stayed and made all the necessary phone calls. To this day, I can't recall one single detail of the meeting, spoken or otherwise, yet I've seen my documentation. Every specific detail had been meticulously recorded. My boss had, of course, taken care of the insurance specifics.

I have never been able to remember driving myself home and pulling into the garage. I have vague, swirling memories of opening the door into the house, staggering across the hallway into the kitchen. My husband looked up from the newspaper he was reading. "What did you do? Drink your lunch?" he jokingly asked.

"I'm sick, Ed. Real sick. I'm going to take something for this headache and go to bed."

Ed was a third shift communications tech manager for AT&T. Having worked all night, I knew he was tired and sleepy so I gave him the seemingly accurate explanation of having the flu. I sure didn't want him catching it, so I downed some Excedrin and crawled into the guest room bed.

Sleep was not to come as the pain was horrible, with no sign of letting up. I felt like I was having the worse hangover of my life, with the added attraction of a volcano erupting inside my head. The sun had parked itself right in the middle of my brain. It hurt so badly! I had a river of flame running through my head. The pain was so intense I couldn't even form a single thought. It worsened by the second, encapsulating my entire being.

After hours of agony, I rolled out of bed and literally crawled down the hallway to the master bedroom. Climbing up on the side of the bed, I cried and begged, and finally got my words out between sobs, audible enough for Ed to hear me. "Ed, wake up, please. I need to go to the hospital."

The mention of hospital broke through his state of slumber as he jumped up and threw on shirt, jeans and shoes.

The pain had gotten so bad that he was on his own, getting me into the car. He was frantic with worry as we headed down the road. "Which hospital?" he asked.

"I don't care," I managed to whisper. There were two in the area, each about the same distance, one due west and the other one north. To avoid the heavy traffic on I-75, we decided on Calder Regional, hoping we could get there quicker. It would prove to be the worse possible choice.

Ed held on to me while he signed me in and gave a verbal description of symptoms to the desk clerk. She said the ER staff would be with us soon. Finding a seat was easy as there was only one other person in the waiting room. Ed sat me down and positioned himself next to me. I leaned against him at first and was soon shifting from side to side, leaning forward and then back. There was no comfort zone. The room swirled around me, the design specks in the tile floor danced in the haze of sunlight and tears.

After a half hour the girl ahead of us got called back. Within a few minutes a woman came in pushing an elder woman in a wheelchair. We heard the desk clerk go through the same litany of questions after being told the patient had a stomach ache. Take a seat. Someone would be with you soon. Ed was exasperated at this point, trying to comfort me, without success, as I moaned and slipped in and out of alertness. He again approached the desk to stress his urgent concern for me and was told that a headache is not an emergency, that I would be seen shortly.

After another 45 minutes, my entire body vanished from my memory. All that remained was the inferno in my head. The fire had now taken on the elements of rocket fuel; the burning was far too painful for me to endure.

"Please, just take me home! I've got to sleep." I thought if I could get to sleep I could surely quash this pain. It seemed as if sleep was the only treatment I could get, especially since the desk clerk already said it was 'just a headache.'

For the third time, Ed approached the desk. For the third time, he was told that I would be seen as soon as possible, that patients are seen according to the nature of their symptoms. "Your wife's condition isn't considered an emergency."

This was unacceptable, and Ed verbally lashed into her, "I wouldn't have her over here for a headache! It's severe head pain! She can't walk! Her eyes are bloodshot! She needs to be seen, now!"

By this time, the lady in the wheelchair had disappeared through the double doors leading to the exam rooms and the room was swirling even faster. Ed came back over and tried to hold me upright, angered and hurt because he was so helpless, frantic that I couldn't even get triaged. My moans turned into quivering sobs and again I pleaded to just go home. Ed cuddled me in his arms and walked me out to the car, but not before stopping by the desk and voicing his anger to the clerk. The ride home vanished from my memory. All I knew at this point was pain. He somehow got me into my gown and tucked into bed, under layers of cover. The pain had reached its threshold. I had no choice but to succumb to the deep darkness of sleep.

Deep inside, I knew the hours were ticking by. How long does it take to get over this? Despite my most sincere efforts, I couldn't outrun this kind of pain. I half woke up every few minutes and forced myself not to move. The slightest movement only sent more flames shooting through my head. The sickening effect of nausea had permeated me by now. It will be out of my system soon, I kept telling myself. Sleep - you've got to sleep.

I battled this intense burning throughout the night. Ed took the night off and spent hours pacing in and out of the bedroom to check on me. My head was a fireball; the pain so horrid I couldn't even cry.

Another explosion of fire erupted, this time sending the lava into my neck. I could make out the streaks of sunshine beaming through the open blinds and struggled through a desperate effort to get up. I hugged the wall and eventually made it into the bathroom. I tried to wet a wash cloth for my face but found I didn't have the strength to squeeze the water out of it. In between flashing bolts of light and haze, I saw myself in the mirror, somewhat distorted, but I sensed the real picture. My eyes were drooping and streaked with blood. I held onto the vanity and cried, realizing at this time, it wasn't the flu I had.

Something worse, much worse. Something so severe I couldn't even make a rational guess as to what it was.

I wobbled toward the hallway again just as Ed was coming out of the master bedroom. I didn't understand the significance of it then, but as soon as he saw me, he turned every bit as pale as I was. Seeing that I had not improved, only worsened, he insisted that we go to the other hospital.

He helped me shower and dress and guided me to the sofa while he hurriedly showered and dressed. Getting in the car and riding to the hospital would never be remembered. There were no words spoken; by this time I couldn't talk. I was literally encased in a world of nothing but pain.

Unlike the day before, Ed got me seated in the ER waiting room before he signed me in. The room was crowded; I saw dozens of people spinning around me. I now had a close, personal relationship with fear, so alone in my world of pain, standing on the edge of a volcano, the earth crumbling away beneath me as the 3000 degree lava flow was pulling me inside.

Ed sat down beside me, offering the only thing he could at this point - open arms and a strong body for me to fall against. It was only minutes later, during this entanglement of fire, nausea and near blindness that I was guided into a wheelchair and rolled back to triage. I drifted in and out until the morphine took control. I could understand that the room was immensely bright and saw the blurry image of doctors and nurses talking to Ed. Their words were nothing but distorted echoes.

During my lapse into nothingness, I had gone through a CT scan. I drifted off again and it was a new pain sensation that pulled me back into consciousness - a spinal tap, as I later learned, not having any idea what was causing the distinct convulsion of pain in my lower back, as if someone was holding a branding iron to my spine, or else, I was having a root canal in my spinal cord, without Novocain.

The doctor was holding out a vial of spinal fluid for Ed and me to look at. He was talking; I could see his lips move; I could hear nothing. I was sinking into another round of blackness.

I later learned that the doctor was explaining that the CT scan had shown an anomaly, suspected to be a bleed in the brain. The spinal tap was necessary to confirm that there was indeed blood in my spinal fluid. The spinal fluid is *grossly bloody,* as the report would indicate.

The doctor gave Ed a quick summary, "We don't have an advanced neurological department here that can handle this situation. I've arranged for an ambulance. Your wife will be lights and sirens to the Acklyn Medical Center. An excellent neurosurgeon, Dr. Samuel Kooper, is gathering his surgical team now. The priority is to stop the bleeding. He will assess your wife as soon as she gets there."

"Can't I ride with her in the ambulance?" Ed asked, thinking ahead that any one of our friends or neighbors would come pick him up once I was stable.

"No, I'm sorry. Not with sirens and the speed the ambulance will be going. You'll hamper the EMT's efforts to provide the care your wife will need during transport; she's very critical at this point. Step across the hall and see the nurse. She has some paperwork for you and she'll be able to tell you exactly where to go once you get to Acklyn."

They don't want me in the ambulance, in case she dies, Ed thought immediately. He was now in a nightmare of his own, it just wasn't pain filled; it was one of total disbelief.

My next instance of consciousness surfaced when I felt the cool, night air on my face. I was in motion, and didn't even try to understand. I was helpless. My situation had rendered me totally submissive to anything.

In reality, I was on a gurney, being wheeled from the ambulance into the hospital. The next time I opened my eyes I saw a blur of people around me - lots of people - doctors and nurses; blue scrubs and green scrubs and white nursing uniforms.

I was immobilized by tubes and probes and IV's and machines, all beeping in a separate set of tones. I couldn't focus or orient myself. I faded quickly this time, not having any idea that *10 full days would pass before I woke up again!*

By the time Ed finished the paperwork at Herritt South Hospital and memorized instructions it was nearly 2 hours later before he arrived.

Dr. Kooper met with him to discuss his initial assessment.

"She has a medium size cerebral aneurysm, which has ruptured. It is about right here," he said, putting his finger on his head to indicate a spot about 2 inches above my right ear. "This has caused a subarachnoid hemorrhage, which is usually always fatal, if not instantly, usually within a matter of days. The rupture is damaging brain tissue every second. I suggest immediate surgery, to clip the aneurysm. That is the only chance your wife has. There is, though, no way to predict the outcome, even with surgical intervention. A lot will depend on her overall condition and health, before the rupture. I'll go over the surgery with you, but you need to prepare yourself as prognosis does not usually lean toward a good outcome."

"What exactly is an aneurysm? How did she get it? She's never had any medical problems." Ed was confused and panic stricken.

"A brain aneurysm is a balloon-like enlargement of an artery in the brain. Once you have one, there is no way to predict if and when it will rupture, but if it does, as in your wife's case, it bleeds into the space surrounding the brain. There are no symptoms until the aneurysm ruptures. Typically, you will experience a sudden, severe headache, nausea, vomiting, neck pain, blurred vision and loss of consciousness, as your wife did."

"We thought it was the flu! This all started yesterday morning! Her brain has been bleeding all this time? For Christ's sake! We went to the hospital yesterday, waited almost 3 hours and she was never even seen by a doctor. She's been screaming with pain."

"I've read the input report, Mr. Magee. She's here now, and will get the best medical treatment and care that we can possibly provide. Unfortunately, the bleeding is causing more damage by the minute. The blood seeping into the spinal fluid puts pressure on the brain and the extensive network of nerves; that causes severe pain in itself. I won't know the extent of damage until I get inside and try to successfully clip the aneurysm."

"Please tell me she'll be alright!" Ed was duly frightened at this point.

"Let me give you the statistics that I know. Each year, 7 out of 100,000 people will have a brain aneurysm rupture. That's approximately 27,000 people per year. 14,000 of those will be instant fatalities. What this means on a local scale is that 1 out of 8 will die before getting to the hospital. 4 will die within a month, even with medical intervention. 2 will be permanently and severely disabled and less than the remaining one will be able to live a normal life. Right now, your wife is heavily sedated. Her vital organ systems, respiration and circulation have to become more stable. Before I get her into the OR, I have to order blood, as she will have to have a transfusion, meet with the anesthesia team and make sure she is stable enough to undergo surgery. Here is the consent form. Please sign it so I can try to save your wife's life."

In a frantic, instinctive act, Ed quickly signed the form and slid it back across the desk.

"If you want to wait in the patient's family lounge, I'll have the nurse come and get you right before we go into surgery. The surgery itself will be a lengthy process, so you'll have plenty of time if you want to get something to eat . Providing she is stable in about an hour, you can walk with us as we wheel her in to the OR."

"Thank you. I'll grab a cup of coffee and be in the lounge. I would like to see her before surgery."

He sat in the lounge, wondering, worrying and waiting.

Should he call my mother? No, he decided he couldn't put her through this kind of worry. He would wait until I was out of surgery and then call her.

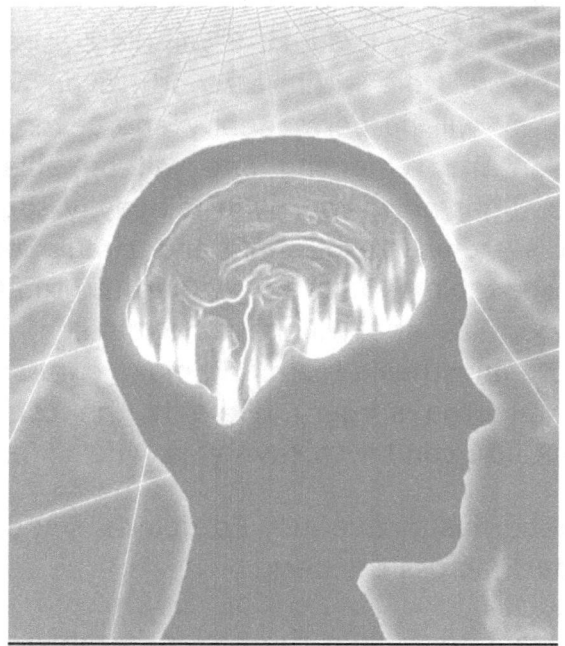

Surgical notes from Acklyn Medical Center

Diagnosis:

1- Ruptured right middle cerebral artery bifurcation aneurysm
2- Right Sylvian fissure subarachnoid hemorrhage .

The situation was discussed with her husband and it was recommended that she undergo right craniotomy for clipping of the aneurysm. Surgical procedure and risks including infection, cerebrospinal fluid leakage, stroke, paralysis, coma and death were covered. Mr. Magee wished to proceed with the surgery.

A four vessel cerebral angiogram was obtained and patient was started on nimodipine. The angiogram demonstrated a 6 X 8 mm aneurysm of the right middle cerebral artery bifurcation

Four units of blood was matched, cross-matched and ordered. BP noted at 91/45. Patient was taken to the OR and placed on the operating room table.

Following endotracheal intubation and general anesthesia, vascular access was established in the form of an arterial line and central line. The patient was then turned and a lumbar drain was inserted without difficulty.

She received Ancef 1 g, Dilantin 1g and Mannitol 50 g intravenously. She was then positioned in the Mayfield pin head holder. The right frontotemporal parietal region was then prepped and draped in a sterile fashion.

A curvilinear scalp incision was made extending from the zygomatic arch to the widow's peak. Scalp clips were applied for hemotasis. The temporalis fascia and musculature were divided with the bovie saw and the scalp flaps reflected anteriorly and secured with clips and Allis clamps.

The Codman perforator was then used to make three burr holes in the right frontotemporal region. A parietal bone flap was then turned using the Midas Rex. The brain covering was moderately full upon removal of the bone section. The lumbar drain was then opened.

The brain covering was then opened in a curvilinear fashion and was tacked up with 4-0 Nurolon. The underlying brain surface was stained consistent with a subarachnoid hemorrhage. The buddy halo was affixed to the Mayfield pin head holder. Self retaining retractors were passed under the temporal lobe section of the brain. Veins in this region were identified, divided and cauterized.

The dissection proceeded under the temporal brain lobe to the olfactory tract and then to the right optic nerve. The proximal internal carotid artery was then dissected out. The dissection then proceeded distally on the carotid to the bifurcation. The middle cerebral artery was followed out into the Sylvian fissure area of the brain.

The Sylvian fissure was then split. At one point in the dissection, bleeding from the anterior temporal branch was encountered and this was controlled with the Bovie bipolar coagulator. Ultimately, the region of the bifurcation was reached. There was obvious blood stain in the region consistent with a hemorrhage. The middle artery trunk was dissected out.

A clip was placed across the artery trunk after administration of Diprivan to prevent another burst. A second clip was placed on the larger of the two bifurcation branches. With this, the aneurysm slackened. The neck could easily be defined. A single straight Yasargil clip measuring 10 mm was then placed across the aneurysm. The Diprivan drip was stopped. Dissection around the bifurcation was carried out, which stopped the bleeding.

Papaverine was instilled about the middle cerebral artery bifurcation. Bits of Gelfoam were packed around this aneurysm clip to bolster it. The area was then irrigated until clear.

The self-retaining retractors were removed. The brain covering was closed in a water-tight fashion with interrupted 4-0 Nurolon. Epidural tacking sutures of 4-0 Nurolon were placed and secured by wire passing through the drill holes. The bone section was returned to the head and secured with four Invisix fasteners.

A #7 Jackson-Pratt drain was placed in the epidural space and brought out through a separate stab incision where it was secured with 2-0 vicryl figure eight suture. The scalp flap was then returned to position. The temporalis muscle covering was closed with interrupted 2-0 vicryl braided suture. The forehead skin flap was reapproximated with interrupted 2-0 vicryl braided suture. The skin was closed with staples.

The lumbar was connected to bulb suction and a sterile dressing applied. Patient was removed from the head holder, extubated and transported to the neuro intensive care unit.

OR time: 6.20 hours
Cerebral blood loss: 250 cc's
Post surgery condition: Critical

One of the OR nurses found Ed in the surgical waiting room and escorted him to Dr. Kooper's office, for an update, or a pretty dismal picture, as it turned out to be.

"I can't give you an exact prognosis. With the brain and especially the hemorrhage, we'll just have to wait and see. We did encounter a couple of unexpected complications during the surgery; a separate bleed and a compressed ventricle. There was a 3 X 3 cm area of damaged brain tissue that I had to remove. There are two major interrelated factors that might surface, both of which could lead to death. She'll have to be monitored around the clock."

Ed sat in stunned silence, trying to grasp the reality and seriousness of the situation.

"Due to the size of the hemorrhage and the extent of brain trauma, I'm concerned about post surgical hydrocephalus - that's a build up of cerebrospinal fluid on the brain, and vasospasms within the brain. We certainly hope she'll be able to bypass these, and be out of NICU in a couple of days. I'll have the nurse come get you in about half an hour, so you can see her. She won't be awake, but you can spend a few minutes with her. While she's in NICU, you can only come in twice a day, for 15 minutes. The nurse will give you the phone number directly to the station so you can call and check on her at any time. Likewise, they will call you if there's any change."

"When will I be able to talk to her? She'll be able to talk, won't she?" Ed asked out of half panic and half excitement.

"No, she won't be able to speak for at least a couple of

days, and that's assuming she will recover, without any complications.   When the anesthesia wears off, she'll still be pretty much a mental blank, because of the analgesic. So, the next couple of days are crucial.   If she makes it through them, prepare yourself for the damage that could range from reasoning difficulties, blindness, speech and perceptual problems, behavioral inconsistencies, loss of coordination, loss of mobility and decreased concentration to constant fatigue. Some of these may be serious and remain with her for the rest of her life. If she survives, she may never walk or talk again.   Some deficits may not present themselves for months, or years down the line. There is no medical way of knowing the exact damage the aneurysm caused. Your wife's prognosis is not favorable, from a medical standpoint. I'm sorry. Let's hope for a miracle in her case."

"But she made it through the surgery. You said yourself that the odds weren't in her favor. Now you're telling me about all these problems she will have – because of the surgery."

"No, Mr. Magee. These damages *might* occur in whole or in part because of the area of the brain that was damaged by the aneurysm and subsequent hemorrhage". Dr. Kooper slid a life size model of the brain in front of Ed and explained, "This is the area of the brain affected. As you can see, the damage was centralized here, in the short term memory, emotion and equilibrium portion of the brain. The damage extended to these areas – speech, comprehension, skin and muscle sensation and concentration. The damage from the aneurysm was so extensive that it affected numerous portions of the functions of the brain".

Ed slowly looked away, not wanting the situation to be real but knowing he understood what he had just been told. His optimism had just faded into oblivion.

The next day when he came in for his allotted 15 minutes, Dr. Kooper met with him again.

Thinking it must be good news, the fact that Dr. Kooper was to be alerted the minute he showed up, Ed was anxious, thinking he was about to find out I would be getting out of Neuro Intensive Care. He couldn't have been more wrong.

"Of the two potentially fatal complications, your wife has both of them - hydrocephalus and vasospasms. That means she has more fluid on the brain and is having spasms in the brain. She's in a guarded hemodynamic condition right now, so I'll caution you before you see her. She looks different than she did right out of OR. There is predominant swelling in her scalp tissue and most of her face is bruised. She'll have to remain in NICU for at least another week while we try to treat these complications. I'm sorry, I wish there was better news to relay."

"But she'll pull through. She'll be alright?"

"At this point, I can only estimate that her survival is less than 5 percent. With the initial damage from the rupture, the hemorrhage and especially now, with the spinal fluid still accumulating in her brain and the vasospasms, she is still in a very critical state. I would certainly like to see her pull through, but as I told you yesterday, hardly anyone can survive this. We're treating her with anti-convulsants to control the spasms, along with meds to reduce the pressure caused by the fluid accumulation. She's heavily sedated because the pressure on the brain is extremely painful. She did rouse this morning when I was in with her. She can't yet respond to verbal commands but she did speak, stating that she was Donna Henley and she was 8 years old. Of course she's not cognizant of anything she does say; the preemptive analgesic, in removing every memory of the pain and surgery, will prevent her from remembering anything for several more days."

"Well, if she's talking, that's a good sign, isn't it?"

"I wish I could give you a more promising prognosis, but unfortunately I can't. She may not make it through the night or the next 3 days. Then again, she may be alive 6 days, a month or a year from now."

"Will she realize who she is, where she is? Will she know who I am? "

"I can't tell you whether or not she will get her full memory back. What she remembers right now is scattered and jumbled around. The brain is running its sensors, if you will, trying to gather what memories it can. It just so happened to be at the third grade stage in her life when I tried talking to her earlier. That was all I could get out of her. That was the only response I got to everything I asked her, that she was 8 years old."

Ed continued his morning and nightly visits. My family came down, even though they too were limited with visitation and had to share Ed's minutes. Ed says I talked to mother and my brother and sister, but unfortunately those memories were wiped away too, thanks to the analgesic. He had started updating my condition on the answering machine at home so that friends, co-workers, neighbors and well wishers would have a current status.

During the next 7 days in NICU, like a zombie, with no real life, just feeding off the habits and motions of life as I used to know it, I created a nightmare situation for Dr. Kooper and the nursing staff. I took out every IV, disconnected every monitor and lined the needles, tubes, probes and sensors neatly on the pillow. I didn't stop there, though. I even removed my catheter.

Had I been conscious, I wouldn't have known where to begin, or even how to attempt any of this.

Since the side rails prevented me from getting *out of bed,* I managed to slide down to the foot end and escape. The dream state of my mind has blurry images; the conscious state recalls nothing.

I didn't get very far as my hospital progress notes later revealed. The nurses quickly captured me and escorted me back to my room, promptly called Dr. Kooper and worked frantically to get me hooked up again. I now had to contend with a Posey restraint.

When Ed arrived, the nurse caught him before he got to my room, to relay the events of the morning, to warn him that I was now under heavier sedation and *restraint.* He went ballistic! Furious over the fact that I was left unobserved long enough for me to have managed that chaotic performance. He was immediately escorted to Dr. Kooper's office, for another medical update.

After being told that there is no possible way to predict the actions of a patient recovering from brain surgery, Dr.

Kooper even admitted that he was surprised that I managed this feat.

"There was no indication that your wife could walk, or was even subconsciously alert enough to move her extremities. Even with the pain meds and lingering effects of the analgesic, she was able to act on her subconscious initiative in a matter of seconds. She won't remember any of this; isn't even aware of what she's doing. This was probably a single act on her underlying impulses, but I ordered the restraint just in case. We're nowhere close to controlling the vasospasms yet and she's still having spinal taps to relieve the build up of brain fluid."

"Isn't that a good sign? Now that we know she can walk?"

"Not really. She's acting on fierce initiative right now. Tomorrow she may try again and not be able to walk. The subconscious mind is responsible for everything she does right now."

"Can you tell me how you think she's doing, in your professional opinion? What her prognosis is now? It is better, isn't it?"

"Only 2 days out of surgery I can't offer you an outcome - positive or negative. For her to survive, she's not even close to being out of the woods. The next couple of weeks are critical. I've seen patients survive the surgery and not have the complications, only to die in a matter of days. Then again, I've had patients I didn't even think would make it through surgery, only to have them go home a week later. Everyone's brain is different, housing most of the healing directives. For your wife, I can only say that yes, her *recovery is possible, but not probable*.

For the remaining week in NICU, I didn't try the escape maneuver again, nor did I even realize I was restrained. I had my daily series of tests, meds and monitoring.

As it turned out, I would never remember a second of the entire 10 days in NICU. My last mental image was the night of my arrival and the partial image of the medical team circled around my bed.

On the 10th day I was moved up to a private room on the 5th floor and the following day I woke up. To the extent that I could, groggy and mentally devoid of time, place and date. If I had been able to actually think, I would have assumed it was the same day I had gone to the ER. So they could extinguish that horrible fire in my head. Was I still in the ER, waiting for Ed to take me home? I didn't know. I certainly didn't realize that 10 whole days had passed.

I slowly scanned the room, taking in my surroundings. I was definitely in a hospital room, connected to a wild assortment of machines, confined by IV's and bed rails. My head hurt terribly, but it wasn't burning, it just *hurt.*

Trying to move proved even more difficult as every inch was in slow motion. With all the wires, probes and IV's, it was impossible. Weak, and not knowing why, I remained in a semi sense of awareness as nurses and doctors flowed into my room. I didn't know who he was, but Dr. Kooper was talking to me, maybe even asking me questions, but I couldn't make his words have any meaning, nor was I able to utter a single word. All I could focus on was my horrible headache.

I drifted back into sleepland and woke up to find several nurses surrounding me, changing IV's, taking blood, inspecting my head and forcing me to swallow what seemed like a dozen pills.

The next time I woke up, Ed and Dr. Kooper were both in my room. I immediately recognized Ed as someone I was familiar with, despite the blur I was still seeing through. Thinking I was still in the ER from 11 days ago, my verbal contribution consisted of, "Home. Take me home."

That put them both on quick, confused alert. They took turns talking to me, explaining the surgery and all the various tests I was still undergoing - spinal taps, angiograms, CT scans. "You will have to stay here for a while longer, you're still very sick," one of them said.

Both my comprehension and voice were playing hide and seek. I could see them talking but couldn't hear a single word. Like watching a movie with the sound muted. The one thing, the only thing I knew for certain was that I was not where I was accustomed to being. I clearly knew that this place was completely different from what my normal surroundings were supposed to be.

They talked for the longest, assuming I was laying there, taking in every word. They could have been discussing the hydrostatic paradox for all I knew.

The next couple of days surrounded me in a drug like drunken state. I was given countless pills and the nursing staff was in my room every half hour, performing their medical duties or transporting me to the testing site on the first floor for yet another scan, angiogram or spinal tap.

Therapists of every genre filled the room every time the nurses left. I moved my arms and legs as if they were made of rubber; mere extensions of my body that would not cooperate in any sense. I floated through each day, with fragments of images and bits of words gathered from the nurses, therapists and visitors. It was all so surreal, not having any meaning whatsoever.

The very frightening part was that I didn't realize this was abnormal. As far as I knew, I had always existed in this hyper state of the unknown. I had always floated through the days. There wasn't one single indication that I knew who I was; no fragment of memory to offer any hint that I had ever even existed before.

I was real, in physical state only. The mental being was stuck at the end of a deep, dark hallway, far away from all that was of critical importance.

All this constant activity going on around me. It meant everything to my survival, it meant nothing to me. On the inside, I was putting up a fierce fight to escape this unknown world. My mind made me try out every characteristic I'd ever known myself, or had seen others exhibit during my entire life. Actions were forced out of me without permission and without knowledge.

The brain healing process is strange indeed. It's a very slow and gradual process. First, you realize you have a memory. Then, you have to get well enough to be able to place that memory into your current being. Not only is it a lengthy process, but a very confusing one as well. Memories don't surface in their entirety. The brain offers up scattered bits and pieces of your life. It's then up to you to sort them out, fit them into the correct timeline and sequence. Every action you manage is in stealth form, invisible to your own awareness. Your body turns robotic, every move a simple act pulled directly from your memory. A hypnotic state of gigantic proportions. Silent commands. Instinct survival. Your mind is blank while your body is so active.

You talk and eat, bathe and respond to the nursing staff, all without knowing it. A wall has been erected between the action and knowledge sections of your brain. Similar to a drunk, waking up after passing out, never able to recall his or her events of the prior evening. Only, this was on a much larger scale. There was no next day 'sobering up' period.

The blessing is that I didn't know if I was sober or inebriated. I didn't even know I existed. Each day thereafter, as the analgesic worked it's way out of my body, I began to recall very small fragments of life. Food, I realized was important but I couldn't understand why, or what to do with the meal trays that kept arriving throughout the day, once I was put on solid nourishment. I later learned I had actually been spoon fed for several days.

I could gaze out my window and have a clear image of the heliport, instinctively trying to figure out what it meant, if anything. I specifically knew what the bright blue piece of machinery was – a helicopter – but that's as far as my memory would go.

I guess in retrospect, if given the choice, I wouldn't refuse the preemptive analgesia. I don't think my mind could endure the memory of all the pain, from my arrival at Acklyn to the day I woke up on the 5th floor. What I did know before the surgery and 10 days later was more than enough memory of the brain explosion. It's just a shame that the 10 day effect of the analgesic not only took away pain memories, but the memory of every other second of those days as well.

The nurses and therapists were careful to chart every word and every action. Many months later, Ed, along with my friends and coworkers recounted their visits with me. None of this would ever become a part of my memory.

A day or two later, I woke up to find that the assortment of tubes, probes, wires and IV's had been removed. I was free! I slid down to the end of the bed and walked around to the headboard, holding on to the side rails for support. I guided myself up and down the side of the bed several times, testing my ability to stand. What should have taken mere minutes took me almost an hour to accomplish.

On one of my trips up and down the side of the bed, I noticed the adjoining bathroom behind me. Bathroom? Shower! I could take a shower. Instinctively knowing what a shower was, instinctively not knowing how to take a shower. I hobbled into the bathroom anyway. At this point, the body was in some systematic operational mode, without involving the mind.

My eyes were in charge - they clearly knew what a shower was. My legs were saying no, no, no, but the directional signal from my eyes was too strong. I had to comply. Actually, I thought I managed the ordeal fairly well, even if it was in a clumsy sort of way. It was probably a very good thing that there was no shampoo available or else I would have surely tried to wash my hair.

I made an awkward attempt to dry off and wrap the towel around me. I turned and noticed the cute little care kit by the sink - lotion, toothbrush and toothpaste.

My body forced me right along as I grabbed a washcloth and began wiping the fog off the mirror. My next action got me confined to bed once again.

I stared in horror at the image reflected in the mirror. My mind was hardly existent but I knew that wasn't me in the mirror. The right side of my head was bald, a huge red and black streak ran from the top of my right eye, curved over my head and ended at my ear. The entire right side of my face was black, blue, purple and orange. The whole 5th floor of the hospital heard my scream. Nurses and aides came running in. Dr. Kooper was paged. I was checked over thoroughly, put to bed, medicated and restrained.

In reality, I only thought I took a shower. No one knows for sure if I even really stepped into the stall. I was satisfied just going through the motions, *thinking* I had really taken a shower. I probably couldn't have figured out the water controls anyway, but I still managed to wrap a towel around my dry body, over my hospital gown.

Every morning and night that Ed visited, he promised to take me home, soon. Family, friends, neighbors and co-workers came in to visit. They blended in with the nurse staff and therapists, just one solid blur. I can only describe it as my brain had literally separated itself from the rest of me. I talked and followed nursing and therapy commands without realizing it. I was put on solid food and was unable to explain that I was not a coffee drinker, and was not particularly fond of milk. Only after the nurse told Ed that I was going back on IV for liquids, did they find the problem. He informed them that I preferred ice water, tea, Kool-Aid, lemonade or Sprite. I sure didn't know how to tell them.

The strong meds along with the analgesic were wearing off. I could feel my brain trying to come back to life, determined to restore itself in full, and realign itself with the rest of me. It started searching, replaying my entire life, giving me a remedial course in *who I am.* The pain slowed me down significantly.

Sleep was accomplished in short bouts after swallowing a handful of pain meds. It was becoming more and more difficult to sleep propped up, but was medically necessary.

There was no explaining the world I was in. Sort of like being in a glass cage, watching life go on around me, in very slow motion. I could understand nothing that was said to me and fought constantly to try and find some words, any words.

I could think now, but just in the present tense although I didn't realize it. Inside, I was trying to cry out to Ed and tell him, "Help me. I'm in here somewhere." Little did I know it would be a year before I made any progress digging myself out of my own brain. While I was searching for myself, inside my own mind, I was subjecting the entire 5th floor nursing staff, Dr. Kooper and his assistants to my character possibilities.

Trying them all. Like trying on every piece of clothing in the entire department store. Too small, too large, too tight, too short, too long. Does anything fit?

I had to go through every emotion the body is capable

of exuding. Not so good for the 5th floor. I tried them all out: crying, laughing hysterically, demanding, screaming, arguing, sulking, refusing to eat, refusing therapy, mockery, impatience, curiosity and rudeness. Then, there was that courteous streak, when I gave all my fruit and candy from gift baskets to the aides.

That act of kindness got me a notepad and pencil in return. I scribbled, at best. I was still trying on personalities to see which one fit the best. I displayed a bit of everything except hunger.

I became extremely mischievous, taking every document and picture off the wall, discarding them all in a corner of my room. Left with bare walls, I counted the ceiling tiles a thousand times and then I got adventurous. I journeyed out into the hallway, taking a few steps in each direction. There I found even more posted and framed documents and photos.

These excursions forced Dr. Kooper to have me moved closer to the nurse's station. Very close. So they could keep a constant eye on me. What they didn't realize is that I could see them also, and even better, see when they weren't there; when they were off dispensing meds or attending to other patients or changing shifts.

The inquisitive mode was sill very active. I had myself convinced that I could escape this place. I had no appreciation of the fact that I was in a hospital. For that matter, I didn't really understand what a hospital was. The first instance the nurse's station was empty I darted off down the hallway and soon found a stairway. In my footies and open back gown, I ran down the stairs, headed for freedom. The door at the bottom was locked and I couldn't place this fact into perspective. I just knew I was trapped. I was probably cold also, since it was February. I shrunk down in the corner between the stairs and door, in disgust, completely puzzled.

It may have been minutes or hours, but the next movement I was involved in was being escorted back to my room. After getting me into a clean gown and new footies I was politely scolded. They were frantic. With worry and the certain reprimand they would get from Dr. Kooper, for not watching me closely enough. They had called a *code purple,* locking down the entire hospital in their search for me. Oh, well. I was still in a fog, unaware of anything I was doing.

With my brain away from the mass of sleep inducing pain meds and sedations, I was a reforming force to be reckoned with. My curiosity now turned to the telephone. Words didn't mean much, but I had an instant recall of numbers, phone numbers. I called every friend, neighbor, family and business contact I had ever known in the past 5 years or so, begging them to come rescue me.

I called my work number about a dozen times a day, each time asking them to send someone to come and get me. Somehow they all seemed to placate me. By quickly calling Ed to let him know my dire intent.

When he visited the next morning, he didn't mind scolding me either. Not that I could comprehend time, but he did tell me the major problem was that so many of my calls were taking place in the wee hours of the morning. Oops. My phone was quickly removed from my room. The nursing staff also taped a big sign to the wall beside my bed saying 'No Phone Allowed'.

I guess curiosity spoke volumes in my case. What could I say? Timing was on my side? The next day I was back in my lookout persona. I was in a state of sheer joy as I managed another escape from my room. Somewhat upset, to the extent I could be, at having my phone removed, I chose to walk off my anger. This expedition led me to peek in every door on the floor - linen closet, nurses' lounge, janitor closet, sterile dressings and the mechanical room.

I did not have the ability to understand that I was in a hospital. For that matter, I had no idea where I was. I just knew it was someplace strange, somewhere I didn't want to be.

The last room I looked in turned out to be a gold mine. It was a patient room, but it was empty. I quickly spotted the phone on the bedside table. Walking over to it, I traced the connection to the wall outlet, abruptly disconnected it, grabbed a clean towel from the bathroom and wrapped up my treasure. Although my body was moving very slowly, in my mind I left the room quickly, in a hurry to get my stolen prize back to my room.

The floor was getting quite busy, so I hugged the handrail, moving very slowly, appearing to be walking, for therapeutic purposes. A part of my daily regime, but with supervision. If caught I probably would have made some excuse for why the therapist wasn't with me. In all reality, I would have been escorted back to my room without a chance to offer an explanation. I didn't see all these people as medical personnel; they were just strangers and I was in a very strange land.

I got close to my room and dashed across the hallway.

Safely inside, I stowed the phone in the closet. Until I was certain my next vital check, therapy treatment, doctor visit and meal were completed, when I was supposed to spend a few hours sleeping. Time flew by. The nurses finished with me for a while and supper was served. Dr. Kooper came in to check me over and Ed made his nightly visit. I begged and pleaded with him to take me home. I got the same response he had been giving me for the past 3 days - *Soon!*

Finally alone, I slid out of bed and got the phone out of the closet, plugged it in and dug the directory out of the nightstand, grabbed my pencil and got started on my project. There's got to be somebody in this entire book that will come get me! I poured through the Yellow Pages, looking for a hint. I couldn't find anything that related to hostage help. I was frantic, knowing I could easily be caught at any time but failing to understand what it meant exactly.

Had I been reincarnated? Was I with the CIA in my former life? The me I really was would have been truly incapable of the sequence of events I was displaying.

I spotted the big BellSouth ad and the light bulb in my head flashed with an idea. I quickly dialed the number for repairs, telling them my phone, my original phone, didn't work. Insistent that they come to this hospital and this room and bring me a phone! I was like a hibernating bear, waking up before the end of winter. Full of retaliatory motion. I poured through the yellow pages, scouring the attorney ads. Surely they could help get me away from these kidnappers! I tried several numbers only to hear the answering machines. I didn't realize it was well after 6:00. I also didn't understand that I had undergone brain surgery two weeks ago.

Eureka struck when I happened on the taxicab section. That's it! I can call a cab to come and get me. I gave no thought to what would happen if they wanted to know my destination. The nice cab man would call Ed and get that, wouldn't he? I managed to get a cab company dispatcher on the phone and relay my plea, that I need to get home. The man seemed nice enough as he asked, "Where are you?"

"In a hospital, I think," I replied.

"Ma'am, I need an address."

"Ummmm. It's a big building. I can look out my window and see a helicopter."

"Ma'am, I still need an address."

I scanned the room and saw the hospital information packet on the nightstand. I found the imprinted logo, complete with address. I quickly read this off to the nice dispatcher.

"Ma'am, that would be the Acklyn Hospital, right?"

"Uh huh."

"You'll need to be at the Park Street entrance in 20 minutes."

"I'm on the 5th floor."

"Ma'am, we can't come up to your room and get you. You'll have to be at the main entrance."

"I can't! I don't know how to get there."

"I'm sorry. I can't help you. Goodnight, ma'am."

ARRRRRGH! I slammed the phone down at the precise split second the nurse entered for a routine vitals check. Needless to say, this phone was quickly taken away!

My head hurt constantly and I couldn't put that in perspective. I think all of my attempts at escape were my way of trying to escape the pain. No matter what doses of pain meds I was given, the pain would not subside. I probably called Ed 3 or 4 dozen times a day. Of course most of my calls went to voice mail because I placed them when he was either sleeping or at work.

I was steaming mad when Ed came in the next morning. I couldn't call anybody. Not even him. I demanded that he get me out of here. "They don't have any medicine here, to help my headache" I kept insisting. "If you won't take me home, at least go get me a prescription for this headache."

In order to appease me so I would rest and not get further agitated, he said he'd go talk to Dr. Kooper and would be right back.

After what seemed like hours later, I peeked out in the hallway, looking for him. I didn't see any sign of Ed, but I did notice the BellSouth man, talking with the nurses. I crept back into bed and waited. Waited for the phone man to put my phone in. Waited for Ed to take me home. Both were going to be great events in my life. I relaxed so easily that I fell asleep.

I slept through all my therapy treatments, visitors and even lunch. The nurse came in and went through her daily routine; the aides helped me bathe and dress into another gown. Dr. Kooper's assistant came in to check my staples and read the chart entries for the day. I was insistent that my head hurt so he said he'd let Dr. Kooper know.

Along with supper, I was given some vicodin and I gladly swallowed it down, desperate to get rid of this headache. All it did was make me nauseous and drowsy. Ed tiptoed in for his nightly visit.

"Hey, sweetheart. How do you feel? I just got through talking to Dr. Kooper. He said he had to give you some stronger pain medication for your head. Now do you understand why you can't go home yet?"

I was so sleepy I had forgotten all about wanting to go home, much to Ed's delighted relief. I fell asleep and didn't even know when he left.

I woke up hours later, to a narrow beam of light streaming in from the hallway. It was pitch dark outside the window and I was begging my mind to hurry and catch me up with my situation. I scanned the room and jolted into my capacity of reality the second I saw the wall plate for the phone. Still empty. No cord and no phone.

The overhead speaker make the nightly announcement that visiting hours would be over in 10 minutes so I knew it was almost 9:00. I head read that on one of the notices I took off the wall. I also knew that Ed had forgotten me again. I stepped out into the hallway, hopeful that I would catch a glimpse of him, talking to the nurse. The only people I saw were 3 or 4 visitors, leaving for the night. As they turned the corner, I clumsily scurried to catch up, racing along the handrail.

As I turned the corner, I saw the elevator doors close.

Elevator? Think, Donna, think!

If I stood there, I'd surely be caught. Change of shift would be due soon, maybe any minute. I stood there, studying the huge gray doors. Instinct took over and I pushed a button with a huge green light on it. Once inside the square traveling box, I panicked. What now?

I looked at the row of buttons and somehow managed to push L for lobby. The next time the doors opened I could clearly see a set of double glass doors across the room, and beyond that, the parking garage. Garage? Cars. Ed's car. My car.

I strolled out into the garage and looked around. For a garage this size, there weren't that many cars, but it looked like thousands to me. It was freezing and damp but I was on a mission. I didn't know make and model but I knew numbers, specifically the number of our license plates. I gave no thought to the fact that even if I did locate one of our cars, I had no keys to gain entry with. And driving would have been out of the question. I ambled around, reading the tag on every car and was, after a while, approached by a security guard. After he asked if I was OK, I frantically shared my plight with him. He graciously offered his assistance. Let's get you back inside and see what we can do, he said.

Finally! My knight in shining armor had arrived! He was going to help me get home.

What I didn't know was that another code purple had been called. I thought I was being rescued, only to find that I had simply been captured again.

The result of this capture started me on an explicit path

to survival, born out of frustration and determination. Everyone was telling me fibs, promising to help me. Nobody was going to help me. I would be stuck in this unfamiliar place forever, without knowing why. Nobody here could do anything about this horrible head pain!

The nursing staff checked me over and the aides dressed me yet again, in a clean gown and new footies. Dr. Kooper came rushing in to check me over as well. I put up no objections whatsoever until I saw the newest piece of durable medical equipment they had obtained - just for me. A new bed. A special bed. An enclosure bed. A virtual cage with heavy netted sides and top. So I could literally be zipped up inside of it. Dejected once again I fell into a deep sleep, totally deprived of any more thought.

The nurse came in before breakfast, unzipped the right side of the bed, checked me over, took vitals and inspected my staples. Good news. I would be allowed out of my *cage* for most of the day. I had the therapists to contend with in addition to blood work and another CT scan scheduled.

After the aides got me bathed and dressed, another aide brought the breakfast tray in. I tried to eat a few bites but my mind was spinning with thousands of arbitrary thoughts. I pushed the tray aside and peeked out into the hallway. I wanted something for this constant headache so I walked across the hall and stood at the nurses' station, leaning on the counter, just waiting. Waiting for somebody to show up.

I stood there in frustration, about to give up and go back to my room when I spotted it. The phone. Stowed in the top of a cart, the cord and cable wrapped around it.

My phone! It had to be. The BellSouth man had brought me another phone! I grabbed it and quickly darted back to my room, stashing it under the pillow. I ran around to the other side of the bed and opened the zipper a mere inch and resumed my place in front of the breakfast tray. Anxious to start my dialing marathon, I jumbled food around with the fork and sipped at my orange juice.

Finally, the aide came and removed my tray. Hurry up, I was silently screaming. I've got things to do before the therapists come in. I've got to plan my escape! I can surely make dialtone contact with someone that will come get me!

Once I was sure solitude was on my side, I poked two fingers through the opening in the zipper. I sawed the zipper with my fingers, centimeter at a time, until I could eventually get my whole hand through. I grabbed the zipper tab and freed myself. I plugged the phone in, jumped back into bed and reversed the zipper process, closing it tightly around the phone cable.

After my litany of calls, I got more promises to rescue me. I fell for it again. In my smoothed-over state, I drifted off to sleep again. The therapists woke me when they unzipped the bed. They allowed me time to stagger into the bathroom with assistance from two of my aides before the series of exercises began. Fearful that I would attempt another escape, I was rarely left alone.

An hour later the therapists finished, the nurse came in to check me over and lunch was served. It was during this meal that I remembered my phone. I reached under the pillow only to find it was gone. Gone!

This was one of those rare instances in life when I gave up. I was suddenly no longer interested in making any calls. My desperate goal to 'escape' just wasn't working out. Besides, I knew someone would come and get me soon. They all promised they would!

The next day was so hectic I didn't have time to think about leaving or even calling anyone. I was so exhausted that I didn't even beg Ed to take me home. I had a CT scan, X-ray, carotid angiography, spinal tap and blood work. I had more pills to take. My head hurt horribly and here I was, trapped in this bed. I couldn't even run from the pain.

After lunch and a nap, a couple of nurses, accompanied by Dr. Kooper's assistant came in and readied my wheelchair. "Time to get your stitches out, Mrs. Magee."

"Can't you taken them out while I sleep?"

"No. We have to go down to the OR for this. It shouldn't take too long. I gave you some pain meds and they should be taking effect by now. That's probably why you're so sleepy.

The staples. All 46 of them. One by one. I grimaced and yelped, screaming every time the steel claws wrapped around each of the metal fasteners. Even with the pain pills, it hurt horribly. I was given even more pain medicine once I got back to my room and quickly feel asleep. The events of the day had taken their toll.

I missed Ed's visit that night, which would have been short anyway as he spent most of the time talking to Dr. Kooper. About my clear intent to escape this prison I was in.

"The brain is a fascinating creation. With all the damage your wife suffered - the aneurysm itself, surgery, fluid build up and spasms, there was no medical way to predict how the brain would respond. I had one survivor that spent 4 days with her knees tucked under her chin because she was hallucinating. Seeing bugs and spiders crawling everywhere. I've seen brain surgery patients throw food on the walls, at the staff and all over the room. The majority of ruptured aneurysm patients unfortunately didn't survive long enough to display any irregularities, but I've never, ever had a brain aneurysm surgery patient try to *escape*! She's acting on subconscious impulses and is not aware of anything. She won't remember any movements she made; any steps she took or any words she spoke. She seems to know that she's in a hospital, but for some reason thinks of it as a prison, a place she's been kidnapped and kept at. She's showing a decline in her anger, and seems to be content even in the enclosure bed. In a few days, providing there is improvement, I'd prefer to discharge her to Acklyn's rehab facility, but I'm really hesitant to send her from one place of confinement to another. I started her on some stronger anti-convulsants this morning so that should help her brain relax."

"What kind of rehab facility are we talking about? She will have a fit once she realized it's not *home*."

"It's a specialty facility that treats only neurological conditions - for example, strokes, Parkinson's, Alzheimer's, brain trauma and post operative brain surgery. The only other option I have is to discharge her to you with home health care. Of course, your house will have to pass medical inspection first, to make sure there are no stairs or danger areas. You can think about these two choices for a couple of days and we'll see how she does in the interim.

Regardless of which discharge, she'll need to take oral meds, and a lot of them, for a few months. These spasms may take a month or more to diminish."

I breezed through the next two days, without causing the slightest disruption. I even recognized 3 of my visitors but couldn't recall their names or our time together. I don't even know if there was any conversation. I complied with all verbal nursing commands and was an excellent therapy patient. The urge to fight my captivity had lost its meaning. The days were so busy I was sound asleep when Ed came by at night.

On a Wednesday morning, I was actually able to shower with the assistance of an aide. After I was dressed in clean gown and bright yellow footies, I had every intention of jumping back in bed and for the first time, turning the TV on to watch some CNN. I walked out of the bathroom only to find my wheelchair waiting.

"Let's get you downstairs for a final set of films and tests," the nurse said.

Final set? I couldn't place the meaning, but happily complied for my ride down to the first floor. Another surprise was thrown at me that day. No therapy. And yet another difference, the lunch was special. No run of the mill hospital food. An actual tray of perfectly prepared low sodium veggie lasagna, corn, rolls and chocolate mousse. I either got bored, distracted or full after a few bites. The aide was duly frustrated but I didn't care. Being nice was nowhere in my realm of capabilities. She put the spoon down and wheeled the tray table cart into the hallway. I knew things were different, but I couldn't fill myself in on the details. My brain was stuck! I wanted answers but even if I had them, I wouldn't have had the capacity to understand them.

Ed, accompanied by Dr. Kooper came in after supper, another special meal of chicken cordon bleu, rice, baked sweet potatoes and key lime pie. This time, my chart would denote that I ate a whopping third of the meal.

Dr. Kooper checked my head, studying every staple scar, every burr hole indention and ended by tracing the circumference of the bone plate I had removed and reattached during surgery. My scalp was still red and inflamed from the staples. He checked my vitals, eyes and ears and then had me do some walking stunts for him. Across the floor, forward, backward, arms out, arms down, arms up, carefully aided by his surgical assistant. He made some notes in my chart and said he'd see me in the morning. Ed and I talked and before I even brought it up, he said he would be taking me home in a couple of days. As long as you do everything the nurses tell you to, he added as a reminder. Of course, he could have been reciting the Greek alphabet and I wouldn't have known the difference.

Ed was at the hospital very early the next morning, telling me he was going to talk to Dr. Kooper again and he would see me tonight.

"With the amount of family members, friends and neighbors that will be available to help, and having a passing medical evaluation on your house, I am going to discharge your wife home. With home health care. She is very unstable in gait and balance. A fall could be fatal. It's imperative that she rest and continue the Nimodipine, 2 every 4 hours. They will be ready for pick up at the pharmacy in the lobby, along with vicodin, percodan, phenergan and Darvocet. You can see which pain med she adapts to best, while at home, and I'll keep it refilled. She'll be in pain for quite a while, sometimes more severe than others. In your discharge packet is a list of things to watch for. I want you to call me if any of these symptoms appear, or if there is worsening of any kind. The home health nurse will be reporting directly to me, so I'll still be monitoring her pretty close. I'll schedule the discharge for tomorrow at 11:00 A.M."

"I've already had a 30 day leave from work approved, so I'll go ahead and start it. I want to be at home with her, until she gets well."

"Now, some important reminders. She can't lift anything, or undergo stress of any kind. No loud noises, no loud music. The least amount of sodium as possible and as much fluids as you can get down her. No over the counter medicine of any kind. If you can close blinds and curtains or manage to darken the bedroom she'll be in, that will be better. She's still sensitive to bright lights. All this will be in her discharge instructions. Any questions?"

"No, I can't think of any. Should I tell her tonight or wait until in the morning?"

"I'll leave that up to you. From what I've seen, her agitated state has somewhat diminished. She can credit herself mostly, for her own survival - her overall health before the aneurysm and certainly her strong, determined character. I am certainly proud of this moment, even though she's still got a very rough road ahead of her. I'm not releasing her from my care until at least December. I don't see any medical reason why you can't tell her this evening."

"Thanks, Dr. Kooper. Thanks so very much."

"You're welcome. I'll check in on her in the morning when I write her orders and they'll be at the nurse's station for you. You'll need to bring her back in 4 weeks for a check up. She'll need to come here for a CT scan first and then take her to my office in the Professional Building across the street."

Dr. Kooper stood, walked around the desk and extended his hand. "Take care of our little medical miracle and I'll see you in 4 weeks."

"Absolutely. Thank you, Dr. Kooper."

Ed came waltzing in my room that evening, and for the first time, didn't grab for my chart at the foot of the bed. He unzipped the side of my bed nearest the door and pulled up a chair. He held my right hand and told me the good news. I'm finally going home.

"You're not well; you're still healing and you have to get plenty of rest. You have a lot of pills to take, but I'll be there to help you. We'll get you better, I promise."

The pain pills I had taken before supper were making me drowsy. I knew it was good that I was going home but I didn't know the difference between excitement and sighing. I drifted off and Ed went home to make sure all the blinds were closed, officially begin his leave from work and grocery shop for anything he thought I might want to eat and drink.

The next morning as I showered with the assistance of

an aide, a couple more aides gathered my personal belongings and placed them on a wheeled cart. Since Ed would be bringing my street clothes, I had to settle for gown attire for a few more hours. Breakfast was served and the nurse came in to do a final vital check and inspection of my surgical scar. She spent an hour reminding me what to do and what not to do. At least I heard her, but my brain had some kind of buffer around it, drastically limiting the amount of words it could interpret.

"You did excellent with the solid foods yesterday, so you need to try to eat that much every day, if you can."

"Ummmm." That was most often my response of choice.

"You can thank your husband and your family and friends that visited. We kept quizzing them about your favorite foods. That was your special treat for getting better, for getting to go home. You've been through quite a scary ordeal and we're all so glad you made it."

"Ummmm."

Ed arrived with my clothes and carted my few remaining belongings down to the car. He had been taking fruit and gift baskets and plants home nightly so they wouldn't accumulate. I think it was because he didn't want me to start throwing fruit at the aides. I sure couldn't eat it, not even really knowing for sure what it was. He stopped at the nurse's station to sign all the papers and go over discharge instructions as I watched from my wheelchair; the aides were busy collapsing my bed.

My journey from the 5th floor began. All the way down to the lobby I was in a state of silence, only half alert, half scared and very confused. The aides waited with me while Ed went across the room to the pharmacy and then to get the car.

Ed opened the passenger door to the car and the aides guided me into the seat and got me buckled in. After a round of goodbyes and take cares, I was headed home.

The sunlight was a whole new sensation and I squinted at the brightness.

The ride home was a strange sensation indeed. The vehicle motion seemed familiar, but different. I could have been on a boat or a spaceship, but then, I was still pretty heavily medicated. It had rained and was kind of cold. The bright sunlight forced me to keep my head bent down for most of the drive though.

Home. I was like a horse wearing blinders, casually being led to wherever I was supposed to go. Ed guided me inside and the first thing I felt was an endearing sense of spaciousness. As compared to my hospital confinement. It was all so eerily familiar but my sight was off, not letting me see the real familiarity. Ed had already turned the living room into my resting zone. The sofa was neatly covered in plenty of blankets and pillows, leaving the loveseat and chair accessible. The blinds were all closed tight, with the only light coming through the arched windows, 25 feet above me.

He later explained to me that he had hidden the deadbolt key to the patio door as well as the key to the gate lock leading to the pool. In my current state, I didn't know what a pool was, but I guess he was afraid I would get in motion and the consequences would be anybody's guess.

He had cleared the huge glass top coffee table and I noticed the bareness but couldn't understand what it meant. I soon found out.

He got me changed into a gown and propped up on the sofa while he emptied the car. I lay there, in total unawares as he loaded the coffee table with bottles of water, glasses of juice and pills. Lots and lots of pills.

He fixed toast and encouraged me to take my pills and eat while he read through the stack of discharge papers.

His latest phone update had informed everyone that I would be home this afternoon and it wasn't long before the house filled up. With friends and neighbors laden with food and gifts. Everyone was talking to me and to each other.

I was high on a mountaintop, watching in slow motion all that was going on around me. My best friends were within three feet of me; they might as well have been a mile away. As a group, they were all on a merry-go-round and I was watching it spin around. My whole world was a circling blur.

Ed took charge and graciously herded them all out, thanking them profusely, knowing they all had my best wishes at heart. It was too much, too soon. My head was hurting badly; the compression was exceeding my threshold. Ed had managed to get the food put in the fridge and freezer and sat back down to resume his reading. That's when the first scare occurred. Ed jumped up and grabbed the small waste bin from the office. My toast and juice would not be digested after all.

I settled back down and moaned constantly. The nausea had really made my head hurt. Assuring him I was as good as I could get for the time being, he ate and made some phone calls while I drifted in and out of sleep.

It would be many months before I could shed this trance-like state I was in. The real world was going on around me, yet I was buffered on all sides, seeing everything through some sort of gray plexiglass shield.

The closest thing to a description would be wearing those drunk driving goggles that the highway patrol use for educational purposes. In a sense, I was drunk from the surgery. Only, it wasn't the kind of drunk you could sober up from. It was like the brain was wearing a straight jacket; blocking it from anything normal, anything real. Everything I had known my entire life was squashed, crushed beneath layers of sutures, gelfoam and titanium.

Every minute of the first several months was spent trying to get free from this locked-in feeling. The pain kept me from succeeding as much as the after effects of the surgery. I still couldn't truly understand that I had surgery; as if my brain refused to remember anything about the entire episode.

I couldn't understand this because the physical restraint I was under made me totally helpless. Even worse, it was with me around the clock. I desperately wanted to jump in the conversations taking place around me but clearly lacked the ability. My talking skills had all been used up on my hundreds of phone calls and now, for some reason, my communicative talents had scurried away, disappearing somewhere in the depths of my brain. It took weeks of searching before I finally found my voice.

I could relate to Ed when I was in pain, yet cold or hunger had no significance. I completely failed to recognize either signal. He said I was much more content once I got to come home. Although in familiar surroundings, I was still pretty much lost. Most of my 24 hours a day were absorbed with pain.

My vision was hazy at best, only permitting me to see things as ghostly images. My walking was limited to a dozen steps at most, just those necessary to travel back and forth to the bathroom. The floor seemed tilted or slanted, as if gravity refused to accommodate me in any way. I was still captive because of my condition but at least I was at home.

I was deeply frustrated – everything was going on around me and I couldn't participate in anything! Couldn't engage in or follow a conversation, couldn't read, write, walk or think. Even worse, I couldn't even express my frustration. Everything in my world related to pain.

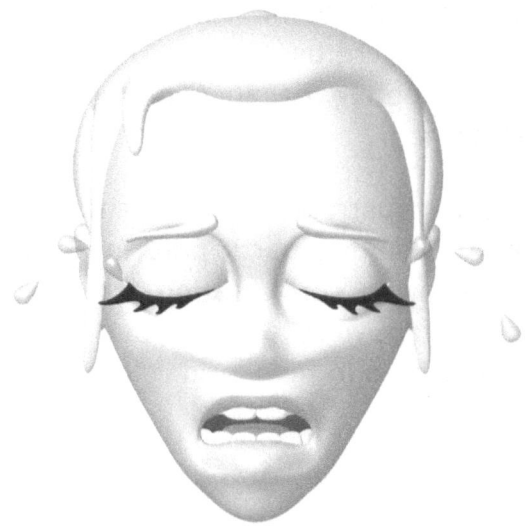

Part Two

Surviving the first year, 2003
Pain, my daily companion
Held captive by my own brain
I used to do that, didn't I?
Hey, I'm on autopilot

Mother and my sister, Kathy arrived early one morning, happy and smiling, trying their best to hide the worry and concern as they hovered about, trying to do anything and everything they could. Ed unloaded their car, full of all kinds of goodies - gowns, footies, housecoats, bathrobes and house slippers. Valentines candy and cookie tins. Then they helped me open all the gift bags that had been dropped off to Ed while on was on my 'brain vacation.' We soon had a floor full of puzzles, cookie tins, cross stitch kits, candles, lotions, sweaters and get well cards. I studied each item as if it was a TV prop on Star Trek. Nothing fit into perspective.

Food kept arriving. It was a generous, wonderful act of kindness, but none of it interested me in the least. There was only one thing that I wanted to eat - chili. I was so adamant about it that Ed and Kathy had to make a trip to the grocery. Back home with the ingredients, mom and Kathy made me a huge pot full, enough to last me at least a few days. It tasted wonderful, and the best part, it was the only thing I could keep down.

Ed had started a spiral notebook so we could track my medication. We went over it a dozen times: look at the digital readout on the clock, every time it showed 2, 6 and 10 I was supposed to take my dosage of pills. He had to remove the caps from each pill container and make new labels, simply identifying each container as pain, nausea, spasm and bad pain. I was very meticulous with recording each one I took. It was a chore that involved no swirling masses of activity going on around me and I excelled at it.

The next afternoon, one of neighbors, a beautician, came over and ever so carefully cut the hair on the left side of my head, so it didn't look so bad next to my bald side. For good measure, she brought me a couple of wigs, thinking vanity still ranked close to the top of my list of priorities.

As it turned out, it was truly a nice gesture after all. I felt pretty good the next day, except for the compression in my head. I sure didn't feel like being confined to the sofa for another full day, so I suggested we all take a ride. Ed, mom and Kathy were thrilled that I felt better so we headed out. Going down the road, we decided to visit a local mall, especially the craft store so we could meander through the assortment of fun projects.

It seemed like a good idea, until 10 minutes later I was hurried back out to the car by Ed. I was nauseated beyond belief. Bad idea. Up and out too soon. But, *I thought I had felt so good!*

That event kept us all at home for the rest of the weekend. As home health would be starting the next day and Ed still had over 3 weeks off, mom and Kathy left to go home and I retreated to my dizzy, moaning world of drifting in and out of sleep.

I had run out of chili and Ed started putting saucers of chicken strips, tuna fish, crackers and Krystals in front of me. Nothing stayed down. Not food, not juice and not even water. Ed called Dr. Kooper on Sunday night. In addition to instructing Ed to make sure I took a phenergan pill before eating, he called in a prescription for a new kind of pill - a sleeping pill. It was imperative that I rest, and more specifically, sleep, he told Ed.

Ed ran next door and got my neighbor, Frannie, to sit with me while he went to the pharmacy. I was so sick at this point I was sobbing constantly, *my head hurt so bad!*

By the time Ed returned, Frannie had added a bowl of water and stack of wash cloths to the coffee table. She was frantically washing my face, wiping away tears and trying to cool me down at the same time.

Between the two of them, I ate a couple of low sodium crackers and swallowed down the sleeping pill. I didn't even know when Frannie left.

I woke and saw the bright digital readout of 1:58. Almost time for the spasm pills, I realized, as I still knew numbers. If we could talk using numerics, I would have probably known everything that was going on.

I made an attempt to sit up which quickly alerted Ed. He had been dozing on the loveseat. After escorting me to the bathroom, getting my pills down me and getting me situated again, I was content to just sit there, propped up, looking around for something to count.

"I'm going into the office to check my email while you're resting. I'll be right here, right down the hallway. How about if I try to find you a movie to watch?"

He turned on the TV and started flipping through the

menu. "Hey! Broken Arrow. You like John Travolta."

Oh, yes. John Travolta. I would like that a lot! I washed my face again and got propped up into my movie watching position. Watching the HBO movie previews before the feature presentation, I was crushed again. The motion made me dizzy and threw me into another vomiting spell. My eyes couldn't keep up with the colors, the bright swirls of movement. My cries brought Ed rushing into the living room.

The next three weeks were spent with me propped up, encapsulated with a constant pressure in my head. I was as human as I could be only when I showered and dressed or the three days Stella came in came in to monitor me, review my pill dosage and bring more prescriptions. Neighbors and co-workers were still coming by with an assortment of home cooked meals and fast food entrees. I made a whole hearted effort to try and eat but every bit threw me into a bout of nausea. And every bout of nausea started the spasms all over again.

I was so sick I cried constantly. I knew I would never be able to endure this kind of pain; the constant compression. The past and present had all become meshed together in my mind. I had a long way to go in order to sort them out.

One night, during an especially painful spell, my mother called. I cried into the phone, begging her to help me, telling her I didn't think I was going to make it. I was convinced the pain would soon kill me. Although normally strong, with a very high tolerance to pain, this was way outside my scope of endurance.

My regional boss called and I relayed the same opinion to him, crying through the entire conversation. Ed grabbed the phone away from me and started explaining his concern to Karl. His wife was a trauma nurse in Chattanooga, and Karl suggested that she call Dr. Kooper to see if I could get transferred to her hospital in east Tennessee.

"I might get her to agree, since she thinks so much of Lana. She's got to have something done; she can't go on like this. I'll never put her back into Acklyn; she thinks that place is nothing but a prison. I can't do a damn thing for her; neither can the home health nurse and it's breaking my heart."

"OK, give me Dr. Kooper's information. I'll have Lana call him in the morning."

No matter how much I wished for relief, I couldn't get my brain to cooperate. Daily conversations with Dr. Kooper always ended with the same instructions - rest and more rest. The brain is still healing and will take a very long time to settle down into its new, allotted space within my skull.

Ed and Lana talked back and forth many times over the next few days. From a medical perspective, it was too harmful to transport me. "The post surgical brain trauma, I know, is very painful. Dr. Kooper is going to have the home health nurse bring some stronger pain meds. She's going back on morphine, Ed," she told him.

"I hope she can tolerate it, Lana. The percocet, percodan, vicodin, demerol and dilaudid just seem to make her sicker. She goes back to see Dr. Kooper next week anyway."

"The morphine will make her sleep anyway. I know she's in a lot of pain with the nausea, spasms and trauma to the brain. Every time she moves her head it probably sets her back a full day. Besides, it's been less than two months since her surgery. The complications have really slowed down the recovery process. Karl will be down to see her one day next week; if you need anything please let us know."

"I will, thanks. Tell Karl I look forward to seeing him."

Stella came the next day and did in fact put me back on immediate release morphine pills. I almost welcomed the many hours of sleep. It was the only time I didn't hurt. The pain was waking me every few hours so I fortunately didn't miss taking any spasm pills. Ed would wash my face and try to force a bite of food down me and I tried to stay awake as long as I could, mumbling through conversations with visitors, hearing the dull echo of Ed's voice talking on the phone.

When he had to leave, to go to the grocery story or pharmacy, I remained propped up on the sofa, staring straight ahead, begging for the pain to please go away. The phone rang constantly; it was just a phantom noise to me. I later learned, other than friends and co-workers calling to check up on me, the medical collection process had started. In less than three months, almost a hundred medical facilities wanted their money; most had not even allowed time for my insurance carriers to pay them. I had full major medical through my group plan at work, and was covered as a dependent under Ed's medical plan through AT&T. The one thing I never considered, or expected, was to be caught up in a medical billing nightmare.

The days drifted by and it was time to go see Dr. Kooper for my 4 week post discharge check-up. After getting dressed, I sat on the sofa while Ed gathered all my traveling necessities: blanket, pillow, crackers, 7 Up, bottled water, wet wash cloths and barf bags.

I was nauseated and sick every mile of the way. My body rejected the very idea of being in motion. I felt instant relief once Ed got us to the hospital parking garage. The cool March air felt wonderful as we walked. Following Dr. Kooper's orders, we went to the hospital for blood work and a CT scan. An hour later we walked across the glass enclosed pedestrian bridge to Dr. Kooper's office in the Professional Building. It was a long walk, because I took baby steps, moving so slow in my world of restraint. Like wearing scuba gear on land. The physical confinement was very frustrating.

While Dr. Kooper was performing his thorough inspection, the lab tech walked in with my scan films and displayed them on the x-ray illuminator. Dr. Kooper finished his exam, walked over and studied the images for several minutes. Ed joined him and Dr. Kooper started pointing out the featured attractions - burr holes, skull fasteners, aneurysm clips, repositioned bone flap and path the saw had taken around my skull.

We then walked across the hallway and got seated in front of his desk while he sat opposite us, my huge file open in front of him. "You're still in the very early stages of the healing process. I talked to a neurosurgeon on staff at Cliffside Hospital, where your boss's wife works and he agreed with me. The transfer would no doubt be detrimental to your condition and there is nothing more they can really to. There's simply no way to speed up this healing process. If more hospital time were medically necessary, I would readmit you. You would basically be getting the same treatment you are getting at home. I think to confine you back in the hospital, any hospital, would agitate you and I don't want to take that chance."

"That makes sense." Ed replied. "Don't you think so, sweetheart?"

I didn't offer a reply because I couldn't; too tired and much too weak to think.

Dr. Kooper continued. "The damage caused by the aneurysm was severe, extremely severe. My prognosis was hovering somewhere between poor and good. The massive amount of complications would have normally been impossible to overcome. You've made it this far, and I know it's been painful, but just think, 7 out of 10 cases like yours don't make it 30 days. You wouldn't have either, without surgery. You would have bled out in another 6 hours. It's very important; urgent, that you keep resting. Even a very slow recovery counts in your case."

"I know. I realize you saved my life. But my head still hurts so bad." I stuttered through tears of sheer pain.

"I'm afraid that is part of the healing process. I wish it wasn't. I have to tell you though, Mrs. Magee, you have to give yourself some credit, a lot of credit in fact. Your tenacious subconscious character and overall good health were partly responsible for your survival."

I had dozens of questions running through my mind;

the effort it would have taken to ask them wasn't there. Captive again. With no voice, just thoughts. When does survival actually begin? The minute the pain stops? The day my memory is restored? The day I wake up and don't have to rely on pain medication? No way could I consider my current status as surviving. I was trapped in layers of pain; an entire galaxy away from being close to normal.

All this talk was making me dizzy. I couldn't get the meaning of the whole conversation to soak in so I leaned back and became a silent fixture. After a couple of minutes, I excused myself and went to the restroom, just outside the office door.

"Even with her slow recovery, she's going to be all right isn't she?" Ed asked.

"I still can't say. I know we talked about this before, when I was leaning toward the medical opinion that she wouldn't make it through the first 24 hours. Now, with all the damage, I still give her somewhere in the vicinity of 5 years, barring any unforeseen complications. Nerve damage will probably overwhelm her physically and I can't begin to guess when that will start happening in a month, a year or 2 years from now. She's suffered an enormous amount of damage to her brain. There is no medical way to accelerate this type of healing."

"If her medical clock is ticking I would like to see her get well enough to make the most of the time she has. I still hold out a lot of hope for her to get better. Is there any possibility of that?"

"Well, on the optimistic side, everyone's brain is different. She may surprise us both and make it beyond 5 years. If she does, it will not be without deficits. There's no medical way to pinpoint survival. This survival rate is so low that I can't make a medical prediction. I don't want to diminish your hopes, but in reality, I can't extend a great deal of hope. Her vitals are improving, but she still has recurrent vasospasms. I'm writing a new prescription for her pain control, Tramadol. Start her on it if after she finishes with the morphine."

I came back in and sat down as Dr. Kooper was writing out a prescription, and still talking to Ed. I was hearing the conversation but it had no relevance. They might as well have been discussing Euclidean geometry. The words entered my auditory canal, but got stuck in the layer of surgical fixtures that were now part of my brain. Knowledge had nowhere to go. It just sort of floated around until persistence let it seep inward, one or two words at a time. Getting placed into the right file cabinet inside my mind was another feat of disdain.

The most frightening part was hearing about damage that I didn't even have yet. Nerve damage. From severed and destroyed nerves; caused by the aneurysm itself and the surgery. *It will be a long time for the extent of damage to manifest itself. Months, maybe even years*, I heard Dr. Kooper tell Ed.

On the plus side, I had made it so far, without complete loss of any one function. In a way, Dr. Kooper explained, the location of the aneurysm had worked in my favor. Forming, swelling and eventually rupturing in the brain section called the Sylvian fissure. One of the most prominent structures in the brain. A divider of sorts, that separates the frontal lobe and parietal lobe from the temporal lobe. Like the median on a highway, except it was the communications center of the brain, the hub of activity, the command post.

For an aneurysm the size of mine, this was the ideal place for it to form. A centimeter in either direction would have permanently removed my ability to see, speak or walk. Since the aneurysm ruptured in the *Corporate Office* of the brain, every sense and human capability was affected, to some degree. In my case, a 20 to 25 percent loss to everything: speech, mobility, hearing, sight, digestion, reasoning, memory and recognition. Damage that is irreversible. Damage that will never get better. The outlook was bleak and dismal. Thank goodness I couldn't fully comprehend it.

Very calmly, Dr. Kooper handed the script to Ed and reminded me to eat as much as I possibly could, keep my head propped up, take the spasm pills for another month, rest and sleep. The head pain will decrease somewhat, in time, he assured me.

Ed and I left for our long trek home. Not only did I have to come back every month and see Dr. Kooper, but starting in a few days I would have to see my personal physician once weekly. Home health would continue for the rest of the year, another 9 months. All this, in hopes of keeping me out of a rehab facility.

How do you cope with a medical atrocity? Especially one you don't know the first thing about? No one in my entire family or circle of acquaintances had any idea what an aneurysm was, especially a ruptured one. We had a basic understanding of brain tumors and strokes, but this? It's one of those life altering events you have to experience before you are propelled into learning about it.

It does give you a deep, profound sense of empathy for any person suddenly struck with diabetes, cancer, muscular dystrophy, heart attack, Parkinson's, Alzheimer's or any other infliction that creeps up without warning you of it's impending attack, forever changing your life. There is no educational path in high school to learn about this; to become educated in the aftermath of handling a medical disaster. Why? It's probably not a general aspect of life. Most of us learn through caring for our parents or grandparents in their elder years. But even that only gives us a vague idea.

You have to fly a plane to know what the pilot experiences, see what he sees, understand wind speed and altitude. That was my frustration point. There were no instructions. The *aneurysm survival guide* didn't exist. My whole life was now like a shooting star. Sporadic bursts of reality. A surprise in the night sky. You don't know what will happen next, nor does anyone else.

For the next four weeks, Ed moved me into the guest bedroom to get me away from the sunlight shining in the decorative arched windows. I was finally able to shower by myself in a clumsy sort of way and Stella had started me on walking exercises. I was talking somewhat better, but sill having to work my way through a hazy, spider web when I walked more than a few steps. I had been off the strong pain pills for almost two weeks, convinced they were the main reason I stayed so nauseated. Ed had been cutting them in half which helped somewhat. I was only half as nauseous for half as long then. I made myself bear the compressing, heavy feeling of pain from my neck up.

It was time for Ed to return to work so one of my friends stayed with me at night. Rita and Janie spent the most time with me, patiently working with me, teaching me the basics all over again. How to turn the deadbolt on the front and back door, tie shoes, open and close window blinds, fold clothes and make sandwiches.

While I slept, they tended to all the housework and routine chores. I was catching on pretty quick, so at least they didn't have to repeat the same group of instructions every evening. I had always been a fast learner; at least that aspect hadn't changed.

My walking sessions with Stella got longer. I opened cabinets, drawers and closets, intently studying all the contents. Trying to figure out how all this stuff fit into my life. The bathroom closet and vanity held no interest. I had a new beauty routine anyway; cosmetic free. Even if I knew what all the bottles, jars, tubes and compacts were for, I couldn't see well enough to make myself up.

Karla, one of my co-workers, had been coming over every Wednesday evening to sort through my personal mail and write out checks for Ed to sign. I watched and learned but concentration of that sort sent my head into a spinning frenzy. She read all my get well cards to me and I vowed to get well enough so I could send out thank you cards. Every detail of each day's events meant so much, yet so little.

It was pretty instantaneous, when I did finally experience a hunger pang. Ed was thrilled silly. I couldn't describe exactly what I wanted so I insisted he take me to the nearby Winn Dixie. An outing other than a doctor visit. Oh boy!

It was an adventure for me and a total hair pulling out

experience for Ed. He pushed the buggy up and down every aisle as I stopped and inspected each box, bottle, bag and jar. My final choices weren't numerous; I pretty much stuck to basics, as I knew them. Banana popsicles, Pop tarts, tomato juice, apples, bananas and oranges. Food that had to be fixed; prepared, totally repelled me. I knew that I used to cook, practically every night, but couldn't visualize the first step in knowing how. I didn't exactly understand the tunnel I was in; the one that wouldn't let me be me.

My new world. Full of pain and simplicity. In less than 10 seconds on that cold January day, I had gone from being healthy and well to being in hell.

Time quickly rolled around for my next check up with Dr. Kooper. It was now three months after the surgery. I got ready and Ed showered and dressed while I gathered my necessities for the trip. He found me in the kitchen, frustrated because I couldn't get the wet washcloths into the Ziploc bags. He patiently solved that problem and put the cake mix back in the pantry and grabbed the box of Saltines I thought I had selected.

Again, we went to the hospital first and then walked to Dr. Kooper's office. First, I got called back to the therapy room, for a quick speech eval. Ed was talking to Dr. Kooper when the nurse escorted me to the exam room. Dr. Kooper was studying my films so Ed helped me up on the exam table.

After his exam, this time, he helped me down and escorted me over to the scales. He recorded my weight and guided me into a chair beside Ed. Positioning his swivel chair in front of us, he started his summary.

"You've lost 31 pounds, Mrs. Magee. That's not a good indication that you're recovering. Are you eating?"

He was asking me? I couldn't answer because I honestly didn't know.

He looked at Ed for an answer. "Everything that falls in the category of real food doesn't stay down. Not even orange juice. She can get about half a Pop tart down and almost all of a banana popsicle, a little tomato juice and some water, when she takes her pills. Crackers won't stay down; nothing I've tried so far."

"You have to start eating. If I don't see a weight gain next month, I'll have to put you on a liquid supplement."

"What is that? Ed asked. "Something like Ensure?"

"That's exactly what I mean. Or else, put her back in the hospital and insert a feeding tube. I know she may not be getting hunger signals yet, or if she is, may not recognize them for what they are, but she has to eat."

"I'll make sure of it. There's got to be something. I just hate to see her throw up everything she tries to eat, although it's not as bad as it was last month."

"I'm going to prescribe some more phenergan. The nausea should be subsiding since she's not taking that many pain meds now. Every expulsion of stomach contents puts her in danger of more spasms, so she'll have to stay on the Nimodipine another month at least. This weight loss is a real concern, though. Since the day of surgery, she's lost a total of 37 pounds, so, whenever she's awake try whatever means you can to get her to eat."

Ed shook his head and agreement and I just sat there listening to them as they discussed me, like I wasn't even in the room.

"Now," Dr. Kooper continued, pointing to the x-ray illuminator box, "the skull is not fusing together as fast as I had expected. Some of that is because of the missing bone particles lost during the sawing process. And, of course, the one dime size section of bone that is missing completely. All of this is affecting the overall fusion process. I'm keeping a close watch on this, and as you know, Stella is checking it 3 times a week, as is Dr. Stoll. It is imperative that she never falls or hits her head in any manner. Other than that issue, it's still very much a wait and see recovery. She's incredibly strong and has a very determined character. I would like to be optimistic, as I'm sure you both would, but it does take a very long time for the brain to heal, especially one that's been through what yours has."

He handed Ed the prescription for phenergan and said he'd see us in another month.

On the drive back home, Ed detoured off the interstate and pulled into Steak 'n Shake. Wow! That jogged a bit of memory. I was excited over the colorful meal photos at the drive up. Ed read the items off to me and I stopped him quickly. Hamburger, fries and chocolate shake.

Ed drove as I ate. Tried to anyway. I got down a couple of fries, two or three bites of burger and a sip of the shake and was completely full. Overwhelmed, actually, as my system wasn't yet adapt to that much real food at once. I stashed the leftovers back in the white paper bag just as Ed was pulling into the drugstore.

"Do you want to go in or wait in the car?"

"I think I'll go in; look around while we're waiting on the prescription."

The first five minutes went well. Ed turned the script in and we started down one of the aisles. He knew from the look on my face and the ghost-like shade of pale I quickly exuded. He rushed me out to the car. So much for my burger, fries and shake.

By the time we got to the house, tears of pain had streaked my face; the throwing up process sent my brain into convulsions, so much so that I demanded the strongest pain pill I had. Sleep saved me once again.

I woke up in the state I was accustomed to when I wasn't nauseated - weak and trying to remove this horrible vice my head was in.

The next few days showed some signs of improvement. Even Stella remarked that I *looked good.* Ed was seeing to it that I had a milkshake in my hand every minute I was awake, so she was thrilled to record my weight at 109.

I felt better than I'd felt in months, and even ventured outside, much to Ed's horror. Just a few steps out the back door, for a short jaunt around the pool. I loved the fresh air and sense of freedom. I moved slowly, curiously and cautiously. I didn't even realize I was walking. It was simply a habit of life. Life from the way I used to know it.

Most of the dizziness began to subside, just leaving the head pain and feelings that were akin to being way down in a deep, dark cave. Every sound an echo, and clearly, I couldn't find my way out.

I still couldn't watch TV but was intent on trying to read. It took all my concentration and effort, but I managed to wade through the stacks of mail left behind after Karla went through it and pulled out the monthly bills.

I discarded the junk and opened the rest, most of which were medical claims vouchers, EOB's and bills. I made neat stacks on the dining room table, adding to them every day. Ed wasn't the slightest bit interested; that chore had always been mine anyway. I had Karla following my normal pattern; putting Ed's mail on the breakfast table and leaving the rest for me to sort through.

I knew I was an expert with anything clerical, basic or comprehensive and was very pleased as I diligently added to the stacks of mail on a daily basis.

Another trip to the grocery with Ed had us both on a dire mission. Find something I could eat. The pickings were thin. Not too many low sodium items for one thing, especially in prepared foods. In the end I settled for V8 juice, pudding cups, Jell-O and more fruit. Besides, we had to reserve room in the buggy for the 5 or 6 half gallons of ice cream so Ed could keep me in milkshakes.

It was Ed that remembered the chili and ran out that evening to Wendy's. It was great. And yes, I did keep it down. So great, that I started having Wendy's chili and a chocolate shake for supper every night. Then I ventured into Krystals and finally pimento cheese sandwiches.

Stella's visits were now only 2 hours long. Thankful that I was finally off all meds except the Tramadol for pain, she focused on my mobility, vitals and scalp scar.

It was time for our monthly trek to Atlanta and much to our relief, Dr. Kooper just shook his head and smiled as I stepped off the scales. "A whole 2 pounds. That's a start in the right direction."

When we got into our review session of Stella and Dr. Stoll's notes, I proudly told him I had started writing thank you notes and signing checks. I explained that I was opening the mail and separating it into neat stacks on the dining room table. He listened intently, though I know I must have bored him to tears.

He had to relent and admit that perhaps I was resting. "The brain, although still healing, is much improved. No matter how good you start to feel, just remember, no driving, no lifting, no stress, no physically demanding housework and no returning to work for several more months," he said, firmly but politely.

The next week was going well, or as I had started saying, *I was doing weller.* The hazy fog was now only half as thick, the sensation of everything being at an angle was beginning to ease, or else I had gotten used to it. I was eating a little more and able to stay awake for almost 4 hours at a time.

It was on a Thursday when I got *the letter* and, within the scope of my daily routine, proceeded to open it. I immediately recognized the gold foil logo of my employer. The overpowering imprint of the 5 story corporate building.

I pulled out the one page letter and read it. And read it again. I was confused and it took 2 more read throughs before I understood the contents. My own employer, specifically the Human Relations Review Board was telling me that my FMLA time had expired. If I didn't return to work within 5 days my position would be filled. I could, however, apply for another position at a later date. I ran into the office and called Karl. He was stunned as well; he didn't know this had been sent to me.

"Let me make some calls and see what I can find out."

Memories flooded my brain! All twenty nine years I had been in the work force. Never out sick before. I worked during high school and through college. I had always worked! I didn't quit working. I got stopped and it wasn't my fault. I never planned on not working!

I was deep in thought when Karl called back. He failed in his attempts to sway *Corporate Mother.* Neither could he understand how I ended up under FMLA instead of disability leave. He guessed they filed my medical situation in a way that benefited them the most. They were remaining firm. If I didn't return to work by Tuesday, I was essentially fired!

I was crushed, hurt, dejected and crying when Ed got home. After explaining the situation, I was further confused that he didn't propel the same tone of aggravation. "You can't work anyway, sweetheart. Not for quite a while. When you get better, we'll find you another job. Besides, I don't think this a company you want to spend any more time with."

"But my license, Ed! I can't lose my license! And what about class? What about my funeral director and embalming schooling? I've got to finish! I can't quit!"

"Look, let's just put it on hold for right now, OK? Until you get better. Then, if you want to go back, I'll support that."

I remained frozen in an emotional, frustrating turmoil until I finally fell asleep. When I climbed out of my stupor the next morning, I showered and dressed and was guided by an invisible force as I worked. Taking all the medical stacks from the table and sorting them - doctor, hospital, lab, pathology, anesthesia, radiology, ambulance, therapy, home health, prescriptions, imaging and ER. By the time I finished, I had over 40 stacks of medical claims, statements and billings.

It was a chore that would have taken the normal person an hour or so. For me, it consumed the better part of four hours. I couldn't comprehend speed anyway, my slow movements were dictated by my brain; my thoughts were the only thing that projected any speed.

I gathered pen and legal pad and took stack at a time into the office, stopping only for Stella's visit and to gobble down a piece of toast and glass of juice.

By Sunday afternoon, I was frantic. The fury had a strange effect though, and I kept it deep inside. I made lists, detailing each facility and service - total charge, insurance payment, co-payment and deductible. I had to stop every ten minutes and massage my head, frantically wishing the pain away as I worked.

By the time I finished, I had added up a total of $226,000 in charges. After deducting the insurance payments from the advice copies, our co-pay, deductible, out of pocket and out of network expenses, my responsibility was showing in black and white as a staggering $62,000.

That couldn't be right. I added again, getting the same figure. I couldn't understand it. I had a seemingly good major medical plan at work, plus, I was covered under Ed's plan at AT&T.

Ed was off work so we spent the evening going over this mess. He saw the major cause of the problem. Over half of the suppliers and services were out of network. In addition we had to pay the out of pocket deductible for both plans. $13,000 each made the out of pocket amount a stunning $26,000. The other $36,000 was relative co-pays, and hefty out of network surcharges, uncovered items and ridiculously high 'we do not accept assignment' charges.

That's the bad thing about independently administered group plans – providers jump in and out of network like Mexican jumping beans on a warm day. Just because some corporate issued printout shows your doctor in network last month has no bearing on their status today!

I could well imagine both of my carriers horribly regretting the fact that I was still alive. Death is cheaper, much cheaper, and health insurance carriers know that well. All too well.

Insurance was my area of expertise and I couldn't make any sense out of this! The hospital was in network. Dr. Kooper was in network. Every farmed out service was not. I just didn't get it! I paid $3200 a year in medical premiums. For all those years I never had a claim, the insurance company was using me, and others like me, for their profit base. And then all of a sudden I have a medical catastrophe and they in turn, *chip in* and pay a contractual amount! To a health care insurer, there is no such thing as *major medical*; they relate only to *major expense*.

It boiled down to the fact that they were ultimately paying a mere 72% of costs. For an average medical bill of $3500, it wouldn't be so bad, to be liable for $980. But, on a large scale, it was a financial disaster!

Their usual and customary geographically approved payments were less than half of the out of network charges. The financial tables had flipped; I was responsible for 70% of all those charges. "We're sunk," I told Ed.

"There is no such thing as a real contract to indemnify. Not even in an emergency situation. What they're telling us, sweetheart, is that you were supposed to get up off the operating table and ask the surgeon, anesthesiologist, lab technician and radiologist if they were in network. Didn't matter that you would die if you didn't have the surgery. They don't care! They quit caring the minute HMO's entered the scene. Besides, they can't get an administration bonus if they pay claims. Think about it. They want us to bear the liability of making premiums and in turn, they want the very minimal responsibility possible with the liability of paying claims."

"I don't think they even set reserve any more, Ed. They just blatantly don't want to pay claims, face it. The minute anything serious happens to you, you're sunk and they know it. You're doomed. A health disaster isn't enough – they have to ensure a financial disaster as well."

"We can't pay this Ed. We'll be broke. Completely broke. I've got to go back to work, whether I can or not! And besides, we haven't even gotten any bills from the last

3 months, since I got home from the hospital. What about all those bills? It's my job and you can't make me give it up" I cried, and ran around the corner, shutting myself up in the guest bathroom. I was crying hysterically and my head was being squeezed so tight I thought for sure the pressure would make it explode. I washed my face, put my gown on and crawled into bed.

Ed came in and tried to console me. "We'll get through this somehow. I'll see if I can pick up some project work on my days off. You just concentrate on getting better, OK?"

I was bright and cheerful on Monday morning when Stella arrived and begged her to reassure me that I was getting better. "You know I can't make that assessment. I can only submit my reports to Dr. Kooper, but I will have to say, you're much better than you were three months ago."

After she left I huddled in the office, going through every file, form, booklet and folder I had that pertained to my insurance plan at work. I read every word on every page. The overall meaning was lost, but deep inside I had a Xerox image of every group insurance benefit I had been paying for. I called Karl and after listening to my adamant statements and protests he had more questions than answers. He would again call my *friends* at Human Resources and call me back.

"You're right, Donna. You do have disability and catastrophic illness coverage. Human Resources is Fed Ex'ing the claim forms out to you today. You want me to drive down and help you fill them out?"

"No, I'm pretty sure Karla will help me. Thanks, Karl. Talk to you later."

I barely had time to make the most important phone call of the day before Ed got home. After forcing myself to remain composed, I got Dr. Kooper on the phone and relayed my predicament to him. After a series of back and forth understandings and agreements, it was as settled as it was going to get. I didn't win my case, but I didn't lost entirely.

Starting the next day, my pronounced deadline date, I could work 3 hours 2 days a week. They can't be consecutive days and I had to be driven and picked up and I could do nothing physical. I called Karl and *told him* that I would be returning to work tomorrow. Then, I relayed Dr. Kooper's instructions.

A half hour later he called me back. *Mother Corporate,* taking in consideration the way they haphazardly handled my absence as a volunteer leave, denied my disability and other insurance payments, gladly consented to my 6 hour work week and confirmed that it would be considered a *return to work.* The bad part, 6 hours would not even pay my insurance deductions. The good part, it would not affect my disability pay, which would be retroactive in lump sum. Besides, I anticipated a fast return to full time. I was almost recovered, almost well. Optimistic me. My hopes were moving at ten times the speed of my body.

I started out working on Tuesday and Thursday, from 9:00 to noon, ready for Ed to drive me the minute he got in from work. That didn't alter Stella's Monday, Wednesday and Friday visits but it did make Thursdays extra long as I would have to go to Dr. Stoll's office before going to work.

The first day back at work was a series of efforts to figure out what I did all those years I spent so much time there. The staff was wonderful, hovering over me for an hour, offering to get me anything I needed; help me in any way. The last two hours I sat at my desk, watching the visual images as they flew by; of all the work I used to do, the documentation, research and consulting.

I was stuck! Somewhere between then and now. The actual act of working had completely escaped my know how. It took the first two weeks to review my file cabinet contents, manuals, mail, rolodex and desk files. It was all so clear in my mind but getting the body to follow through was complicated indeed.

By the third week, I had a firm understanding of all the policy audits I *used to handle.* Karl visited and we all worked out a plan. The staff would continue handling my consultations and leave the intricate policy research to me.

We figured out that I could excel at anything that didn't require movement. All it takes is that first step..... I worked more slowly than before but was extremely methodical and precise. My 3 hours quickly turned into 4 and 5 hours as the staff had overwhelmed me with some very complex cases; batches of policies from the 1940's and 50's.

It was kind of relaxing, combing through the old policies to ascertain a starting point. It was endearing to see the simplistic way things were done way back then.

It was, by most counts, a very natural transition. I had again become expert in tracking down these old companies as I worked diligently, batch by batch, until my body simply shut down. There wasn't much of a warning either. My mind just rather quickly shut the door on the thought process. Time to go home and collapse. It was never a problem getting one of the staff to run me home, besides, we had half a dozen company vehicles at our disposal and I lived only minutes away.

My next visit to Dr. Kooper was quick and painless. For the first time in months, I didn't have to undergo the routine scan. He checked me over, still concentrating on my head for the longest. The consultation in his office was still mandatory.

"I trust that you're not overdoing it at work?"

"Oh, no. I don't have a choice anyway. My brain lets me know loud and clear when it's time to quit. Then I go home and go to bed."

"Good. You still need plenty of rest. Your brain is still healing, and although I hope not, complications could surface at any time. I'm cutting you a break on the weight issue. No gain, but there hasn't been a loss, either."

He then explained to us that he had scheduled me for a cognizant reasoning assessment. It will take a few hours; you'll like Dr. Banchly. She's pleasant, professional and thorough. You'll need to be at Herritt South on Friday morning at 10:00. I'm faxing orders for blood work, EKG and CT scan before you see her at 11:00."

"What the heck is a cognizant reasoning assessment," I asked him. I had never heard of such a thing.

"Let's call it the 3 R's. It will tell us how well your brain is doing with Remembering, Recalling and Reorganizing information and memories. Dr. Banchly can give us a thorough assessment of any underlying damage."

All I could do was exude a heavy sigh and say alright.

Returning to the very hospital that was responsible for the ER triage doctor saving my life invoked a queasy feeling. The staff practically rolled out the red carpet for me. Aides and nurses hovered around, expressing their well wishes, glad to see me doing so well. *Glad to see me still alive.*

The activity was overwhelming. Name tags and faces started dancing around, interrupted by the flashing effects from the overhead fluorescents. I was back in my shroud of fog. Back in zombie land. I was wheeled into the lab and imaging departments. The heated blanket was my sanctuary, protecting me from all the activity, the crowds. My brain hadn't yet learned how to handle that much stuff going on around me. It frightened me terribly.

Dr. Banchly was everything Dr. Kooper said, and more. She was so very kind and soft spoken as she talked to me, getting an overall feel of my mental status, carefully explaining each and every challenge I would have to go through.

To this day, Ed shakes his head in amazement as he remembers me sitting there and so easily rambling off all 50 states, the last 12 Presidents, counting backwards from 100, by 7's.

I was then moved to a table and given a kids 100 piece jigsaw puzzle that depicted a jungle scene. Dr. Banchly set the timer for 30 minutes and prepared to watch, taking notes of my ability to concentrate. Eleven minutes later I was done with the puzzle.

While she made notes, we were treated to wafers and juice. The puzzle was moved aside and replaced with a rather large coil bound book.

Things got really difficult at this point. As she sat next to me and turned each page, I was to study the picture and tell her what was missing from each one.

I was rational, so very rational deep inside my brain, but so confused on the surface. If it's not there, how do I know it's missing? Each turn of the page only frustrated me further. Who on earth would notice one missing reindeer from Santa's sleigh? Or figure out that the calendar page didn't have any numbers on it? Or that the smiley face clock was missing its hands?

After 30 or 40 pages and not one single keen development, we took another break and tried a new task. It would prove to be the most simple, yet challenging of all. Nine blocks, with a vivid geometric design on 3 sides; once assembled the 4th side would depict a boy holding a balloon. Dr. Banchly was kind enough to reset the timer twice. The last time it sounded, I casually pushed all the blocks onto the floor.

It simply wasn't workable, not for me anyway. Ed thought it was too much for me, in one sitting, and voiced his concerns. Dr. Banchly insisted we forge ahead, instructing me to sit in the leather wingback chair and relax. She had a 'set' of general knowledge questions to ask me.

"I can't think any more," I protested.

"Just answer them the best you can," she softly instructed.

She first asked me what day of the week I was born on. My brain no longer had the means to search for answers; I could only reply with spontaneous words as I grabbed at bits and pieces from deep inside.

"It wasn't Friday" I spurted out instantly. She looked at Ed and he admitted that, yes, that was correct. I wasn't born on Friday. June 20, 1954 happened to be on Sunday, Father's Day that year, to be precise.

Question: "Who signed the emancipation proclamation?" Answer: William Seward

Question: "Who was ordered to shoot an apple off his own son's head?" Answer: Johnny Appleseed

Question: What might you add to peanut butter, making a popular type of sandwich?" Answer: bread

Question: "What is the motto of the United States?" Answer: America

There were 50 questions in all, but these were the ones that she and Ed discussed. I was still fuming over the 9 piece block puzzle. The last feat of the session seemed simple enough. I was situated back at the table with a drawing pad and markers placed in front of me.

"Draw anything you'd like to, anything at all," she politely instructed.

I picked up the blue marker and started drawing away. She and Ed talked while I drew.

"She has a long way to go, still, and I think Dr. Kooper may want to repeat this in a few months. The amazing thing is that she's either way off base or extremely brilliant. It's interesting, indeed, at how her brain is reforming."

"She had me beat naming the Presidents and states. Maybe she just can't remember how to do simple things yet? You suppose?"

"That's what is so amazing. She got Johnny Appleseed confused with William Tell. I can't mark her wrong for saying bread instead of jelly. The motto question - well, it seems like the encyclopedia in her brain just picks a select few bits of knowledge and discards the rest."

Dr. Banchly paged through her notes and came to a particular notation she had made. "This is something I have never seen before - William Seward *did* sign the Emancipation Proclamation - along with Abe Lincoln. Seward was the Secretary of State at the time! Probably less than 3 percent of the population know that! So, I'll send my report to Dr. Kooper and we'll go from there."

She came over to inspect my masterpiece. After studying it for several minutes, she carefully picked up the drawing of my boat. So appropriately named the 'SS Headache' I had printed on the life preserver - my ship in the middle of the deep blue ocean, all alone, anchor cast, just stuck out in the mass of water, waiting.... just waiting.

Ed and I left and he insisted on stopping at the Cracker Barrel. I was tired, depleted of any enthusiasm until we got seated and I remembered the huge assortment of vegetables they offered. I ate heartily, convinced that I'd surely gain 5 pounds and make Dr. Kooper very happy.

By July my work load had frightfully escalated. I didn't mind the tedious attention to detail. I actually excelled at it. It was with natural ease and ability that I perpetuated spread sheets, applying fundamental strings of algorithms necessary for each type of insurance, for each individual client. I could easily overwrite the embedded code, to allow for policy administration costs and inflation, so the family could know, to the penny, what the funeral cost and death benefit would be.

I lucked up every once in a while and had the privilege of assessing flawless policies through excellent companies. I beamed with excitement when I saw an Allstate, MetLife, Nationwide or United of Omaha policy cross my desk. My work schedule had now grown into 4 days a week. Stella had changed her schedule, coming in the afternoons but on the plus side, I was getting better. Finally!

Once I got my backlog of policy audits under control, I delved back into the computer arena. I wrote programs so I could log every client profile. When bored, I put together procedure manuals, keyed and converted them in perfect PDF format.

I became so proficient with the pc, something I would have never attempted before, that Karl had me a new laptop, docking station and desk monitor delivered. They were soon followed by a new laser printer so I could start assembling my procedure manuals for the entire division.

I was ecstatic! I finally felt useful! Eventually I was troubleshooting computer problems for the entire building. My A type personality had finally kicked into full gear.

Thinking I had better take advantage of it before I went back into brain lockdown, I tackled every grueling, tedious project I could. When I was at home and woke up in the middle of the night, I scuttled into my office, flew through DOS and located all hidden integrals in my personal computer. I took a pretty in-depth voyage into my hard drive and had a brainstorm one night, thinking it would be pretty cool to send Ed a quick little hello.

I suddenly, distinctively remembered every programming lesson, calculus class and DOS command from my 1978 course in BASIC. As technology advanced, I realized that hacking was just a paraphrase for programming. It took several attempts, but I was finally into Ed's computer at work. I searched for his email account provider. Outlook was so easy to conquer, especially the 1995 version. I opened my own AOL account and sent a cheerful message. I smiled and sat back, ever so proud of myself. Proving to him that I was getting better.

At exactly 2:10 A.M. the house phone rang. I glanced over and saw from the distinctive 775 number that it was Ed, calling from his desk. He got my email!

I cheerfully answered and he nervously asked, "Sweetheart, are you, by any chance, on the computer?"

"Yeah, I can't sleep. Why?" I asked, smiling secretly.

"What in the hell are you doing?"

Yikes! He didn't like my surprise? "I just wanted to say hi."

"Well, miss smarty pants, I just got a call from

corporate security. A breach into our system, traced back to my home phone line! Get off the computer! Now! Before I lose my job! I've got to figure out some way to tell these jerks that my wife is recuperating from brain surgery and accidentally hacked through their firewall."

"Well, okay" I said quietly. I didn't know how to explain that the curiosity side of my brain didn't give one single thought to the fact that I might just be doing something wrong. I was just practicing to be smart again, I thought.

Work volume and the concentration it demanded was the only way I could run from the lingering head pain. At home, I had to constantly invent things that demanded my total concentration - anything detailed and time consuming. I was such a dismal failure at anything simple. My one day off was spent writing checks to pay medical bills. Making no progress. The lump sum disability and catastrophic illness payment went right back out; my employer quickly claiming 6 months worth of insurance premiums first.

By the end of July, I had gone through our entire savings account as well. All $43,000 paid out to medical providers. We had no choice. The mail continued to overflow with even more medical bills. They wouldn't stop, not with the current, ongoing treatment. Both insurance plans combined, at best, were paying out $537.00 for every $1000.00 in claims. I was working simply to make a dent in medical costs.

The Fourth of July arrived and there was a huge community party we had always attended. I was adamant about going this year as well, at least for a while. I was right in the middle of the activity, chatter and music but felt they were so far away. That cushioning effect presented itself because of the crowd. The voices turned to echoes, the hollow sound of my own voice wasn't the least bit familiar.

The effects from the partying would be my ball and chain for a very long time. The picture perfect string of text in my mind began skipping and bouncing around before falling out of my mouth in a scrambled arrangement. Harder to explain was the fact that by all outward appearances, I seemed fine. Just fine.

My July visit to Dr. Kooper was not at all what I expected. Back to the hospital first, for blood work and scans. Then to his office for my exam. He came in with my 4 inch thick file, placed it on the desk, sat down and started scanning the pages. He explained that he was reviewing the notes from Stella, Dr. Banchly and Dr. Stoll. His face gave us no indication whether or not he was pleased or concerned.

My trip to the scales did indicate a 1 pound weight gain. Back on the table for a head, neck, arm, leg and eye inspection he took vitals, jotted the results down and said, "Your blood pressure is erratic. Has been for the last 3 weeks. I'm pulling you back out of the work force until we can get it under control. You will never admit it, I know, or might not even be aware of it, but you're overdoing it. Your job may not be physically demanding but the mental toll is too much."

"I don't think it is, at all. And besides, I dropped out of mortuary school, at least for now. All I have is simple office work."

Somehow during the healing process I had become quite blunt, giving no regard to the terse expulsion of my words.

The nurse brought in the film and placed it on the illuminator. Dr. Kooper walked over to study it. Ed and I just looked at each other and he had to point out, "I tried to tell you. I knew you were overdoing it. Listen to Dr. Kooper. I agree with him - you need to quit work."

I was overwhelmed by my sudden inability to communicate. Crushed. I was unable to tell him, make him understand that *I had to work!* It was the only thing I could do, in fact. And besides, the medical bills were not going to get paid if I didn't work.

Dr. Kooper returned to the exam table and inspected my head again. "Because you can't have an MRI, I'm going to get Dr. Stoll to set you up for a contrast image session. This will take about 2 hours, at a specialized imaging center, so I can get enlarged images of your brain. There's no need to worry, I just need a closer look, to make sure there's nothing going on in your brain that would cause this fluctuation in your blood pressure. This is less invasive than subjecting you to another angiogram."

I couldn't take each separate sentence he said and have a clear understanding of its meaning. I was so limited as to how much I could focus on at once. Despite his entire parlance of words, my mind remained focused on his earlier words *I'm pulling you back out of the work force.*

"You're still a long way from recovery. The overall healing process, especially in your case, could take years.

You're not totally free of complications yet and I want to be able to locate and head off any potential problems, but for now, rest is imperative. We certainly don't want those spasms to surface again. Dr. Stoll will schedule the contrast scan and have the report and films sent to me, so I'll see you in a month."

I called Karl that night and relayed Dr. Kooper's orders. He understood from a personal standpoint but from a business outlook, he was livid! I looked over at the latest stack of medical bills and had an instant plan, which I quickly relayed to Karl.

There! It was solved. I would simply revert to my 6 hour work schedule. Ridding myself of 24 or 25 hours and 2 whole days per week was the same as pulling myself out of the work force, wasn't it? I thought so. I had to at least work through the end of the year, keep my insurance coverage, as pathetic as it was, and make a dent in these medical bills. Then all would be OK. Stella's orders were calendared through December 6th and besides, Dr. Kooper would be releasing me from medical care in December; the end of the year, surely.

Ed relented, mainly because he didn't want to see me upset, half because I was insistent that *I was getting better!*

My contrast image scan was scheduled a couple of weeks later. For the first time in over 6 months, I had to remain lying flat, while the 72 images were captured. It was horribly grueling but I endured; I just wanted it over with. The radiology staff was excellent, covering me with heated blankets and coming out from behind the big glass window every couple of minutes to check on me.

I readjusted to my 6 hour work schedule, again selecting Tuesday and Thursday for my easy 3 hour days. Dr. Stoll ended up prescribing some pills to lower by blood pressure. I felt weak all the time and probably couldn't have worked longer even if I wanted to.

The following month was a jungle to crawl through. Seven months after surgery and I was jolted awake with pain. My neck, left arm, head and stomach were being pounded with a steady stream of fireballs. Ed called Dr. Stoll and was told to get me to his office right away.

After a pretty quick exam, Dr. Stoll sent me straight to the hospital. It was crazy. For 2 months, I felt alright, except for the constant headaches and in just an instant I was being burned up from the inside. My blood pressure had climbed to 178 over 72. Scans and tests revealed even more surprises. A blood clot in my left arm and an enlarged kidney. I was immediately admitted to the hospital. Dr. Stoll and another doctor came in later that day.

"This is Dr. Anders, a urologist. He's going to talk to you about your kidneys. Your blood clot is superficial, and your blood pressure seems to be much better. Now, let's get your kidney taken care of,"

I said hello to Dr. Anders, Ed shook his hand and thanked him for coming in and the medical discussion began.

Kidney stones. Several of them. In both kidneys. And the stones have ruptured. Dr. Stoll had conferred with Dr. Kooper. Neither felt that I was stable enough to endure surgery. "It's the long way around a routine condition, but we can at least keep you monitored with a constant IV drip and oral meds, to hopefully flush the stones out. If we don't have any luck in a few days, we'll have no choice but to surgically remove them, especially if they get buried in the kidney walls, but that would be a last resort, given your condition and the probability that you're not strong enough to endure surgery yet."

It was going to be a really boring few days for me. Ed spent a couple of hours with me after he got off work in the mornings and another few hours before he went in to work at night. He brought me magazines and crossword puzzle books and on the third day, instead of getting to go home, I did have to have surgery; ureteroscopic stone removal. I had to stay another day but at least my kidneys were no longer inflamed, searing with heat. The right one seemed to be the real problem, manufacturing minuscule stones on a daily basis.

Despite his concern that nerve damage was the major culprit, interfering with the daily operation of my vital organs, sending false signals to my kidneys, he agreed to release me with discharge instructions to see Dr. Kooper the following week.

Six days later Ed and I were back in Atlanta at Dr. Kooper's. After the normal and routine exam he ushered us into his office.

"All of the organs, more than likely, will be affected by the nerve damage to some extent. The frustrating part is not being able to predict what organs will be affected, and when. I'm going to start you on a prescription for Neurontin. It will hopefully lessen the severity of pain and slow down the damaged nerve signals.

"Will it make me groggy?" I asked.

"Not physically. In essence, what it will do is slow the nerve signal speed down so that your fragile organs won't feel the zaps of pain as severely as they are now. You can still take your Tramadol or Darvocet if you need to."

I was feeling pretty good during August. The fatigue remained, a dear companion to the head pain, but from all outward appearances, except for the disfigured right side of my head, I did appear to be well.

So well, in fact, that I suddenly grasped interest in a new project. Driving. I imagined it would be like riding a bike; you just don't forget how. I backed out of the garage and went down the driveway; up and down, up and down. Then, I ventured out into the street, to the end of the cul-de-sac, circled around and came back. I was fearless, stopping to talk with neighbors that were outside. Oh yes, I was much better.

Pulling back into the garage posed a little bit of a problem, though. I misjudged the opening and allowed my left fender to come in direct contact with the garage door frame. I was petrified, so I left the car and went into the house. Ed would know what to do when he got home. Besides, I thought my *drive* went well.

"The good news is that you didn't dent your car, just some white paint transfer that I can probably get off. The door frame is splintered a little, though, just a little. I can probably get Smitty to help me fix it. Don't worry about it, OK?"

"OK. I guess I'll just have to leave the car in the driveway and you can pull it into the garage for me, on days I go to work. At least I can still drive," I boasted proudly.

"Sure, sweetheart. No problem."

Another checkup with Dr. Kooper and I admitted to him that I was back at work, 2 days from 9 'til 12:00. Prepared for a scolding, at the very least, I was surprised when he just suggested that I stay on this schedule. Especially with the blood pressure, blood clot and kidney stones you just went through, he reminded me. "Whatever you can do to limit your physical activity will coincide with my orders. I need you both to give this all due consideration." He then escorted us across the hall to his office.

"I've studied the contrast films. The midline shift of your brain is not self correcting. This is the reason things seems angled and off balance to you. This is also the reason you lose your balance after standing or walking for a few minutes. And yes, before you ask, the aneurysm did cause this; more specifically, the swelling of the brain, and the surgery itself."

"You mean, her brain is not centered in her head? Is that what you just said?" Ed asked.

"Well, in raw language, yes. Time may or may not, in your case, Mrs. Magee, allow a reverse shift. I would say probably not, with the amount of trauma and the small void from where the damaged brain tissue was removed."

"So, she'll be OK as long as she doesn't ever play tennis or jump rope or ride a bucking bronco - stuff like that?"

"As far as immediate problems go, yes, that pretty much spells it out. The nerve damage we've talked about before still makes it a wait and see process. As much as I'd like to give you good news - even great news, I just can't. The balance, vision, brain pressure and occasional loss of speech are conducive with this condition, and part of the overall survival. I think you should continue doing what you're doing. Restricted work hours, lots of rest, plenty of water, 3 meals a day, and no stress. How are you doing with Percocet, Vicodin, Tramadol and Darvocet?"

"I give her half of one if she needs it, or if I'm at work she'll take a whole Tramadol. Some days she doesn't take any pain pills at all."

I did feel pretty good, if you don't count the constant head pressure. My last thought every night was to please wake up and have it be gone. It was a futile request but I did manage to jump back into the tedious work details. I flowed through the audits, spent hours on the phone tracking down old insurance carriers and neatly documented all pertinent details. Most exciting - I was now driving myself to and from work.

I was so *mind strong* that you couldn't possibly convince me that I was *physically weak*. At my insistent urging, Dr. Kooper reversed his orders in October and let me add 2 more days to my schedule - 'short days at that' he advised.

I was finally able to handle all aspects of my job - even the personal consultations and funeral pre-arrangements. I had a surprise visit from the CEO, who wanted to personally honor and recognize me with awards for my outstanding, flawless attention to detail with the policy and procedure manuals I had put together.

Deep inside, I thought this was just their way of trying to make amends for inadvertently putting me on unpaid FMLA and disregarding the disability leave. I played along, expressing my appreciation and continued the dedication to my work. By the end of the month, I was offered a promotion. A huge promotion. All this corporate attention should have been so exciting, but I lacked the ability to recognize the glory. They did accomplish the feat of convincing me that I was recovered and eventually I fell right into their enthusiastic and complimentary world.

The years I worked for them, before my brain exploded, I had traveled quite a bit. To regional offices for meetings or the other two corporate owned funeral homes in Georgia that I maintained an office in. Every six or eight weeks I had traveled to North Carolina or South Carolina for a divisional meeting.

Ed and I spent the entire weekend discussing the promotion. Karl, his boss and I sent dozens of emails back and forth, addressing every possible problem as well as recognizing every benefit. My capabilities were never an issue. Ed was concerned about my durability.

But, *I would be in charge* of all 3 insurance audit divisions in the whole state. It would be my sole function to bring the other 2 sites up to the standards I had set at my main office.

Grief relief, as I called it. Training, coaching and ensuring licensure for all employees in my region. The only problems were the trips to NC and SC. Ed solved that issue. He would juggle his schedule at work and drive me to those meetings. He could take his laptop and work from the hotel.

An even more comforting issue was the fact that Corporate was being extremely generous. For my weekly trips to north Georgia, I would check into the local Holiday Inn Express instead of trying to drive back home after working. Besides, Dr. Kooper had strictly forbidden any night driving. My peripheral vision was practically non-existent anyway. And, even better, I could get these dreaded medical bills paid and hopefully start rebuilding our savings.

All went well for a couple of months. My check ups were trouble free; Stella was only visiting one evening a week and I was feeling more and more human every day; my focus being on work, being productive and getting some of these horrid medical bills paid.

It was in the middle of November that I was scheduled for a 'house call.' Death was imminent for this woman's mother and her fragile state wouldn't allow her to come into the office. Reviewing the driving directions she had given me, I guessed it to be about 20 miles away from my home base. It was early afternoon when I pulled into her subdivision.

I sailed through the meeting and was deeply aware of my true compassion and the reality of death of a loved one that this woman would soon be facing. In between a natural outpouring of tears and comfort, intricate details were discussed, selections made and insurance policies were handed over.

It had started growing dark as I backed out of the

driveway so I paused for a moment to recite the reverse directions. After an incredibly long half hour on Highway 20, I started to question myself. This can't be right. It can't be this far. I turned around and backtracked, looking for some familiar structure to jog my memory. I ended up back at the subdivision I had left an hour earlier.

I tried again and still failed to find my turn off. I had no choice but to pull over and call Ed from my cell phone. Giving him a very detailed description of my surroundings provided him with more than enough information. He guided me home, staying on the phone with me every mile of the way. It was such a huge step backwards for me that I never told Ed just how terribly frightened I was. Neither Dr. Stoll nor Dr. Kooper would ever be able to explain why my mind chose this particular time to shut down.

I dreaded my November check up with Dr. Kooper. I had lost even more weight. Shoulder seams on my clothes almost reached my elbows. Armholes exposed half of my rib cage and I could only wear pants with belts or else they slid right down over my hips. I had to delve into my collection of blazers to hide my shabbiness.

As it turned out, I hadn't lost any more weight. I just didn't fully realize that size 6 and 8 clothes were much too large for my size 2 body. After his exam, Dr. Kooper was split between two opinions. He was concerned that I was working too much; yet he thought this was the best healing process for me, especially since there had been good reports - blood pressure stable, no more seizures and I was only taking a Tramadol less than 3 times a week.

I did take Thanksgiving week off. We dined with our closest friends, another childless couple, and spent the day relaxing. With the exception of the holiday meal, I was hard at work, altering what skirts and pants I could. Since it was nearing Christmas, Ed took me to the mall for a clothes shopping spree, so between what I had altered and the new clothes, I thought I had plenty to do me until I gained my weight back.

My family and I ended up shipping Christmas through UPS; I couldn't travel and didn't want them to upset any family time, just to visit me, so we spent hours on the phone. December was routinely my slow time at work anyway, so I did get to rest quite a bit.

I had made it through a whole year, almost. I still missed the alacrity of my former life, the stamina and endless list of physical capabilities but was hopeful that next year I would start to show significant improvement. From the outside, things were looking quite well. I moved through each day without any real complications. Of course, my days were only 10 hours long, at best. From waking up, getting showered and dressed, working, returning home, attempting supper, sorting mail, paying bills and handling some household chores. Normally up at 7:00, at work by 9:00 and back home at 3:30. By 5:30 or 6:00, I was completely useless. My mind closed down and took my body with it.

From the inside, I was still held captive. That inbred and academically learned series of personal and professional mannerisms would not fully materialize. I knew, deep down, that I was - used to be - capable of so much more. Capable of cramming in a personal life after the work day ended. Dining out, movies, bowling, tennis, swimming, shopping, outings with my friends - they were now things I could only remember and no longer take part in.

I was so determined to outrun this shroud of inclusion my brain had seemingly latched onto. The real me, so very badly, wanted out!

Most frustrating was that I couldn't begin to explain this to anyone. Just because I *seemed alright* it falsely led everyone to believe I was healed.

It was like opening a textbook and placing it in front of a blind person. They look like any normal human being. Until you realize they are blind. For me, that was exactly what it was like. No one could see inside my head and understand that I was slow, very slow, in the thought process; that everything around me was slightly out of focus. Sounds and voices were often muffled. My body tried to remain in the here and now but my mind always had other plans.

Even more complicated to explain were my actions. When I wanted, needed to smile, it took my brain a long time to send the proper instructions, so whatever expression was the easiest to exude is what I displayed. Most often was an expression of surprise, no matter the circumstance. Anything other than work related issues put me at a great disadvantage.

My social skills were deeply hidden, maybe they had disappeared altogether. I didn't realize that I lacked this ability. The perfect flow of my thought process to the natural manner of speech or action was interrupted. Social graces formed in my mind but skipped like a broken record on the way out.

The cognizant therapist would later explain to me that

the brain was having a terrible time coping with all the damage. That, more than likely, without the sheer strength and determination of my acquired and learned character, my brain would have shut itself down completely.

As it turned out, determination was one of my strongest and most sufficient assets. It almost had to be since the avalanche of medical collection calls had started. The first call almost sent me back to the hospital for certain as the blatant, cold hearted woman casually called from Acklyn, asking for an immediate payment of $68,229.53. I tried explaining that it sounded like my secondary carrier had not been billed. Didn't make a difference to this vulture. She called several times a week, insisting and demanding that regardless of any outstanding insurance claims, the balance was my responsibility. In the first place, she needed to be talking to Ed. Technically, he was the one who signed all the medical treatment and consent forms. And besides, I wasn't about to make any payments until I saw remittance advice forms from both insurance plans.

The fortunate part was that I slept through most of the steady stream of calls, grateful that Ed utilized his inbred northern bluntness on the ones he answered.

Part Three

Crawling through year two, 2004
Hello, meet your new self
Up jumps the damage
Personality makeover without consent
Disruptions in year three, 2005

Ed and I were looking forward to my December visit with Dr. Kooper; when he would release me; when he would tell me I was better, much better. I was excited at the news I would get. Hearing that I had recovered! A personal, physical accomplishment; a mental reprieve from constant medical bills.

I could feel the gradual batch of changes but for some reason, didn't dare pause long enough to give them any due concern. I just wanted out of this medical nightmare I was in.

Dr. Kooper stunned Ed and I both. No, he wasn't going to release me. Home health was discontinued; no more treatments approved by my insurance carrier. Monthly check-ups would now be quarterly; visits to Dr. Stoll would now be monthly instead of weekly and I had to have a follow up cognizant session with Dr. Banchly.

"Most of Dr. Banchly's concern is the erratic thought process. Especially since you managed to be completely inaccurate, partially right and exceptionally correct - all during the same assessment. What we're mostly concerned with is the nerve damage; the path neurons have to take in order to process thoughts. This next session will hopefully give us an indication of the extent of damage, as far as cognizant and processing skills go, in everyday life, outside of work."

Ed and Dr. Kooper talked on while I remained fixated on the x-ray image of my skull. Pieced together, like a broken dish, the series of cracks so noticeable. I sneezed, instantly getting Dr. Kooper's attention.

"Probably catching a cold" I muttered.

He checked my eyes, ears, nose and throat and asked "Did you have a flu shot yet?"

"Dr. Stoll gave me one a couple of weeks ago. He said if I do get a cold to call him, that I had to have an injection."

"He was adamant that she not take any over the counter cold medicine." Ed said.

"It's imperative that you never, ever put a decongestant in your mouth. Never. And you're probably not going to find any cold medicine that doesn't contain a decongestant. If your cold worsens, call me or Dr. Stoll. You will need an injection."

"What is the big deal about decongestants anyway?" Ed asked.

"They rank right up there with MRI's. Both have fatal consequences. Decongestants would instantly constrict blood flow to the brain; a death sentence in her case." He continued examining me - blood pressure, pulse and temperature and went over to the desk to write in my chart. I got down off the exam table, ready for our normal walk across the hallway to his office. He asked me to have a seat beside Ed. I had preferred to stand in the corner and lean against the wall but I did as I was instructed and sat down.

"Your temperature is up a little bit. Let me go ahead and have the nurse give you a shot while you're here. It will make you sleepy, but will help ward off this cold. Your immune system is much weaker now, understandably so, and you're probably much more susceptible to colds."

I was so groggy by the time we got home I crawled into bed, clothes and all and slept for hours. It was Friday, so I would have all weekend to rest.

The next 3 months sailed by. I fell into a work routine without really planning it, working 10 or 12 hours on Monday, Tuesday and Wednesday. I made the schedule adapt to my reasoning as I would have 4 whole days to rest, not counting the 2 trips to N.C. or S.C.

The impractical side of this was that I was spending 2 of the 4 days in bed. So tired all the time. Blocked in on all sides, physically, as my mind stayed in a speed warp. Thoughts flew through my brain so fast that I failed to notice the one single command, *slow down!*

Because I didn't recognize that one warning, my brain quickly pulled the plug on my endurance.

The two days at home that I was able to basically function, I spent hours in the office, going through medical bills I hoped so desperately would be ending. A new year had started. I shuddered with fear as I realized what that meant. Another $26,000. out of pocket. For the most part, we were self insured, or under the all new consumer driven health plan. Where the consumer drives the train of financial medical responsibility. Our savings had been depleted last year. I had no choice but to keep working just to pay for medical care.

After a few weeks of keying the medical statements into my spreadsheet, I was depleted of any optimism. I watched the subtotals turn into a staggering $32,000 and it was only April. Even with a federal tax refund of $9000, it would take every cent we *didn't have.*

Ed and I discussed every possible solution. To drop me off his plan and only indebt us for my $13,000 out of pocket sounded good, but Ed thought if I got real sick and had to quit work, I would have no insurance and we would be in worse shape than now. It was crazy alright, with both of us working and earning pretty attractive wages, the usual savings allotment was now going to health care! We discussed every feasible option - even selling the house. The solution was clear! I absolutely had to get better.

There was only one thing left. I really had no choice. I had to call our home town bank, our personal banker at First Community Bank. They had been incredibly professional and super friendly, always before, with our mortgage and various car loans. It humbled me greatly to make this call, but I was overjoyed at the outcome. All I had to do in fact, was call. I sensed it in Philip's voice. Once you're a bona fide customer, you're a real part of their *community!* They do back their expert banking with individualized understanding. With a financial plan now in the works, my worry abated tremendously.

Less than two weeks later, the loan papers were signed, the money deposited into our account and I spent the entire weekend writing out checks.

With that aggravation put to rest, I could focus on real life - work and getting better.   It was such a relief to be paying out $415.00 a month to the bank instead of our average $3200.00 to medical bills. The medical facilities were paid; the horrid, terse, demanding phone calls would end; collection attempts before I had even received a billing copy in the mail.

By June, I felt exceptionally well. So well, in fact, that Ed and I took a 3 day trip to Chattanooga. The Riverfest was going on and Ed's favorite entertainer, Delbert McClinton, was the featured performer. During our stay, we took in the Choo Choo and Aquarium as well. It was a splendid time, one I welcomed immensely.

I had kept putting off my next session with Dr. Banchly and vowed to Ed that I would call her and schedule it soon. In reality, I was terrified of knowing the outcome, so yes, I procrastinated. And besides, Dr. Kooper had not mentioned it last month during my check up. He had, however, ordered another round of contrast scans for me, so I figured I would deal with the imaging session and Dr. Banchly on the same day.

It was the middle of July when the bottom fell completely out. I had only been at the office for a couple of hours and my body was suddenly screaming with pain. I felt an instant rush of nausea. My right leg, stomach and neck were turned into soaring infernos of heat. I cleared my desk of work in a half hour span of very slow movements. Then, I prayed for the strength necessary to drive myself home.

Ed was in the master bedroom, asleep, since he had worked all night, so I gathered a pillow and blanket and carried them out to the sofa. I took a Tramadol and crawled under the cover.

I woke to the sound of my own voice, moaning in agony, with Ed wiping my face with a damp cloth, asking over and over, "What's wrong? What hurts?"

My entire body had exploded this time, from the inside. All of my organs were on fire, being mangled, as if they were being sent through a shredder. Ed rushed me to the ER and I just remember being on a gurney, rolling down a hallway, seeing lights overhead, frantic with pain.

Whatever they gave me for pain must have worked wonders. I woke up in a private room, saw Ed sitting in the chair watching TV and felt the confinement caused by the ever so familiar IV's.

"Hey, sweetheart. Welcome back. How do you feel?"

In my half groggy state, I tried to sit up and asked to please go to the bathroom. "I'll get the nurse. Be right back. Don't move."

The nurse helped me maneuver *Henry, the IV pole* into the bathroom. I grabbed the chance to wash my face and try to remember how I ended up hospitalized. I was getting better! This couldn't be happening!

I was put back to bed and some familiar faces came in, the nurses that had prayed for me so frantically during my aneurysm, and greeted me so warmly when I had my first session with Dr. Banchly. I was trying to ask Ed what I was doing here, but a couple of neighbors trickled in and I lasted only about 2 minutes with them before I fell asleep again.

The busy commotion of the morning shift change and breakfast tray delivery woke me. The nurse came in, checked me over, changed my IV and said the doctor would be in soon.

I was eating my toast when Ed walked in. After a gentle kiss on my forehead he said Dr. Stoll would be in soon.

"Why? I'm going home! *Aren't I?*"

"Let's just wait and see what the doctor says, OK?"

Dr. Stoll bopped in, greeted us and started comparing the current monitor readings to those last recorded in my chart.

"How are you feeling this morning?" he asked, as he moved the stethoscope around my back and chest.

"Just a little groggy. I'll be alright once I get home."

"I'm afraid you won't be going home today. You had another blood clot in your left arm; a superficial thrombosis we treated last night. The stomach and legs are a little more serious. Your left kidney is inflamed and enlarged again, due to a pretty good size stone that can rupture at any time. You have a calcium build up in your pancreas as well, and even more serious, your potassium level is well under normal. That's what one of the IV's is, to get your potassium level back up. Dr. Anders will be in to talk to you about your kidney. He'll be the one to arrange your discharge, depending on his treatment plan. I've spoken to Dr. Kooper and he may have some orders of his own; let's see how you progress through the day, OK?"

"What caused all of this, Dr. Stoll? She was fine one minute, and then, *bam!*"

"This is in Dr. Kooper's area of expertise; on initial assessment, he seems to think this may be the beginning signs of serious nerve damage. The internal organs aren't getting the full set of instructions they need in order to work properly. We've seen indications of that all along; gradually, with the lapse of hunger signals and sudden inability to speak at times; the sporadic seizure episodes. For right now, the potassium is the most urgent problem."

"So, this is like a minor glitch, something that can be fixed?"

"I don't see any reason why not. An adequate supply of potassium is being infused back into her and Dr. Anders will get her kidney all fixed up. She may be laid up a while, though, but she'll be fine" he said, giving me a reassuring smile.

Dr. Stoll left and I let out my usual sigh of disgust. Ed tried to comfort me, pleading with me to be patient. The potassium has to be put back in the body very, very slowly. The latest round of pain meds was making me drowsy so Ed went down to the cafeteria while I slept.

I woke up as lunch was being served. Still disgusted with my state of confinement, Ed had to plea and prod me to eat. I managed the broccoli and roll and had Ed slide the tray table away from the bed. I was just so tired and sleepy that eating proved to be too much work.

Dr. Anders woke me up the next time, taking vitals while the nurse recorded them in my chart. She checked my IV's and quietly left while Dr. Anders greeted us and explained the findings from yesterday's CT scan.

"There is a large stone in the left kidney causing the kidney itself to be grossly enlarged. Since the stone hasn't ruptured yet and providing your potassium level gets restored during the night, I'll be doing shockwave treatment in the morning, to blast the large stone into very tiny particles so you can pass them. We'll get another scan this afternoon to make sure the kidney has responded to the IV antibiotics. You'll have some papers to sign, Mr. Magee, so stop at the nurse's station before you leave and I'll see you in morning, Mrs. Magee. You won't get anything to eat or drink after 6:00, so try to eat all of your supper and get a good nights sleep. As far as I can tell now, you should get to go home late tomorrow afternoon."

Ed thanked him and came back over beside the bed, his dejected, helpless expression saying he wished he would be going through this instead of me.

The nurse staff woke me at 6:00 A.M. to escort me and 'Henry' into the bathroom, then got me dressed in a surgical gown and wheeled me down to OR. Ed was standing at the OR entrance talking to Dr. Anders as I rolled by. The nurse stopped the gurney long enough for Ed to kiss my forehead and tell me he'd see me in a couple of hours.

I'm glad I wasn't privy to Ed's conversation with Dr. Anders. Surgery may have had to wait for my blood pressure to return to normal. Dr. Anders explained that there was a chance, *just a chance,* that the procedure may damage the kidney tissue. It was highly possible because of the size and shape of the stone, that the blasting would send shards of the stone into my kidney wall.

I woke up several hours later, back in my room and clawed my way out of the drug induced fog. Ed cheerfully greeted me, saying the surgery went well, except that I had to have a stent put in, to keep any of the stone fragments from getting *stuck.*

I did get to go home the following day, with antibiotics and a new friend - *Sherman,* the bright blue stent, that would remain inserted for 3 weeks. Great. I still couldn't lie flat down and now I couldn't sit straight up so I had to resort to every bad posture position in the book. I leaned and slumped out of sheer necessity.

Ed spent hours on the phone talking to Karl, updating him and insisting that I wasn't coming back to work for at least three weeks. And that was only if Dr. Kooper didn't have any bad news for us, pending his assessment of the symptoms that sent me to the hospital in the first place.

I got put on an actual medical leave this time, not even upset that I would be missing work.

I felt pretty good about a week later; got as used to 'Sherman' as I was going to get and had long ago learned to live with the dull ache that encompassed every square inch of my head. The occasional stings in my right leg were annoying, but thankfully they didn't last long, striking suddenly, like a hot flash of lightning, then vanishing.

I accompanied Ed to the Winn Dixie on Saturday morning. I guess the kidney stone bout had one positive effect as Ed just shook his head in amazement while I loaded up the buggy with popsicles, ice cream, fruit, Green Giant frozen vegetables, apples, bananas and oranges.

By the following weekend, I was doing even better. Ed had received his annual bonus from AT&T and scooted me off to a nearby mall, treating me to some clothes that actually fit. By this time, I couldn't even shop at 3,5 & 7. I was now wearing a girl's size 12. It was horribly embarrassing to search through girl's clothes, but I managed to find several mediocre skirt sets. To make our trip complete, we did find a nice assortment of size 2 slacks and small tops in the Paul Harris store.

The following two days had me confined to bed again. Instead of getting better, I took a downward turn. Ed called Dr. Anders office and was told to bring me right in. I was a mess by this time, sitting up on the exam table, weak and feverish.

After an hour of taking blood, running a urinalysis and going through an ultrasound, Dr. Anders gave us the bad news. A cyst in my right kidney had ruptured. I was full of toxin. I had to have immediate treatment.

Back to the hospital; my home away from home, for another long date with 'Henry.' The nurse assured Ed that I would sleep most of the night with the pain meds Dr. Anders had ordered. "Go home. Get some rest yourself. We should start to see some improvement in the morning," she told him.

Surprisingly, I did feel better the next morning. Ed came in first, followed by Dr. Anders. The infection was severe, but caught in time.

"Can I go home?"

"No. Not for a few days. You'll be on this antibiotic drip for 3 days, but I do have some good news. We can get that stent out tomorrow. If your potassium level and toxin level are managed, you can probably go home the next day. Let's just rest and get you better, OK?"

I had no choice but to rest. Not that I felt like doing a whole lot anyway. Ed brought me in a batch of crossword puzzle books, a few friends stopped by and the nurse was in and out every hour, checking or changing out the 6 hour drip bags. Dr. Anders did take the stent out and I was looking forward to going home on Friday.

Ed was supervising me, making sure I ate all my supper on Thursday evening when Dr. Anders came in. He greeted us, opened my chart and sat in the empty chair next to Ed.

"I hope you're writing out my discharge orders," I half joked.

"Yes, you can go home tomorrow, Mrs. Magee. You have a small surgical procedure to go through first, though. I have it scheduled for 3:00 tomorrow afternoon, and then you'll be discharged."

My eyes closed tight. I was crushed. This can't be real. This is not surviving! I heard Ed ask "What kind of small surgery?"

"You're going to have a PICC line inserted. It will be attached to a monitor and feed antibiotics into you around the clock. You've had 3 days of infusion, your potassium level is now normal, but you've got another 3 weeks of antibiotic treatment to go through. With the PICC line, you can continue the treatment at home. I know you want to go home, your insurance company wants you to go home, so I'm setting up home health to visit you every day, to flush the line and refill the antibiotic."

"My insurance already stopped home health care." I remarked.

"This is a whole new medical situation. They have to approve it for the necessary 3 weeks."

"Between both major medical coverage's, they should cover it!" Ed stated emphatically, then asked, "What exactly is this PICC line? Does she *have to* go through more surgery?"

"As I said, it's a rather simple surgical procedure. She'll be taken into the OR and given a sedative. The doctor will insert a small thin tube into a vein in her elbow and guide it up through her arm and into her chest cavity. It will come to rest just above her heart. She'll be able to feel it but it won't present any physical pain. The antibiotics will be infused through a pump, housed in a carry case that she'll wear in a sort of backpack. The line has to be flushed with saline every day. The nurse will start her visits on Saturday and I'll see Mrs. Magee in my office in 3 weeks, to remove the line."

Me, Ed and our new house guest, the little black pump case, left the hospital Friday night about 8:00. We got me situated on the opposite end of the sofa, where my left arm and the tubing and pump case would dangle freely over the edge.

Karl called, concerned at first, then frantic because I still couldn't return to work. They had hired 3 people, out of necessity, on a trial basis, one at each location, to handle some of my job duties, at least, until I did get to come back to work. When I return, I could keep them on as assistants, provided I trained and supervised them.

I was too agreeable, not the slightest bit interested in discussing my job. I used to care, so much. What I didn't realize was the simple fact that I was no longer able to care.

Confined again. I felt so burdened with the monitor strapped to my side, dangling a 3 foot long section of tubing that sent the liquid into my vein. Ed helped me with my new method of showering the next morning, as I would have to endure it for 3 weeks. A bath, actually, sitting in the tub with my back to the faucet, left arm hanging over the side. The only way we could figure out how to keep it dry. Much more cumbersome was the fiasco of washing my hair in the kitchen sink.

Marilee showed up Saturday afternoon with instruction guides and cartons of syringes, saline, vials, bandages, IV bags and an IV pole. Once she and Ed got everything in the house, they had to count every single item and I had to sign for them. She had insurance forms and authorization forms to be signed. The last was the insurance billing authorization. My insurance company had only approved home health IV treatment 3 times a week! The line had to be flushed and a new supply of antibiotic hooked up *every day!*

"That's insane" Ed said. "First they tell us how long she can stay in the hospital for this treatment and now they're limiting the very treatment they said could be done at home."

There were only 2 choices. For the remaining 4 days a week, Ed had to learn how to flush the line, hook up one of the IV bags of antibiotics, or he would have to take me to Dr. Ander's office and have it done.

After walking us through the 15 step procedure a half dozen times and actually flushing the line and replacing the fluid with a replacement vial she had brought with her, Ed and I were both pretty confident that he could handle the 15 step treatment.

For two hours the next day, we read through the instructions again and again, reviewed all the notes we had taken, identified each separate piece of medical equipment and tried to remain confident.

Though paranoid, we both decided it was something we had to do. Besides, it would cost $73.00 out of our pocket, each time I went to the doctor's office. That equated to $292. a week; a staggering $876.00 for the three week duration. The last thing we needed, especially with me out of work again. My paltry disability pay was barely keeping my insurance premiums paid.

It was nearing 6:00 Sunday night. We had no choice. We had to do this. Ed seated me at the breakfast table and stood the IV pole beside me, hung the saline bag, clipped off the line and opened the clamp for the cold fusion of fluid. The flushing was easy enough. We both breathed a sigh of relief.

He removed the IV bag, attached a new set of tubing for the antibiotic and clamped it off as I watched intently. Count to two. That's how long it took for the antibiotic to begin entering my bloodstream.

In an instant - everything went drunk wild. The room was spinning rapidly. Blood was pouring out of my arm, covering my gown and filling the kitchen floor. Ed was on the phone screaming to 911 while holding on to my arm, trying to stop the bleeding.

I fell, slowly, and kept falling - backwards. A thousand volts of electricity were passing through my body. I could see an image of myself projected way off in the distance. I was floating backwards, like looking through the wrong end of binoculars. My image, getting further and further away; smaller and smaller.

Ed was trying to hold me upright and keep a dish towel wrapped around my arm. He managed to slide me half on, half off the sofa as the EMT crew came rushing in. My blood pressure was 190 over 90. I was fading, slipping into oblivion.

The ambulance took me away while Ed gave a frantic explanation to the neighbors who had come running over.

Leaving our neighbor Frannie in charge of locking up the house, he jumped in his car to head to the hospital.

When I came to in the ER triage unit. Frannie came walking in, a look of fear prominently displayed. "Hi, neighbor, how are you? Ed's talking to the doctor. He gave me these clothes for you. I'll help you get changed. The doctor said it would be alright." She pulled a navy pajama set out of the bag she had and I managed the ordeal of sitting up on the side of the bed.

We both darn near died of shock when I pulled the cover away. The entire left half of my gown was covered in blood. We managed to manipulate 'Henry' and get me dressed.

Putting my bloody gown in the bag she beamed, "I can get this washed out; it'll be good as new."

Ed and the doctor came in the room. Frannie gave me a hug and kiss and made her way out of the room.

Ed stood beside the bed and rubbed my arm as the ER doctor spoke. "You've had a severe reaction to the antibiotic prescription for the PICC line - the gentamiacin. Did you know you were allergic to it? Do you have any other allergies?"

"I've never had an allergy in my life; I've never even heard of gentamiacin."

He asked dozens of questions. Could I possibly be allergic to the latex, in the gloves? No, I had the gloves on, not her, Ed explained.

"Please tell me it wasn't something I did! I'll never get over this! If I did something wrong! That damn insurance company! They have us doing medical procedures to keep from paying claims!"

"Calm down, Mr. Magee. Let's go over everything you did, step by step, once again. Take a deep breath and slowly tell me everything, in precise detail. Take your time."

I was beginning to think Ed needed to be in the ER bed more than I did. And then I became scared. For Ed; for the guilt he must be feeling. We both went over the instructions. There was no way he did something wrong. I followed along as he explained his steps in vivid detail.

The doctor concurred. Ed had followed the directions precisely. We had no way of knowing I would have a reaction to the antibiotic. An almost fatal reaction, had Ed not been so quick to seek EMT intervention.

He had Ed drive home and bring back a bag of the liquid antibiotic. More blood was collected and more machines were hooked up to me. Blood loss had been significant; was there any damage to the heart? Or the brain? The ER doctor worked frantically, especially after learning I was post craniotomy. An MRI was out of the question so he excused himself to call Dr. Anders, leaving me to battle the confusion.

Ed returned with a box full of our PICC line supplies including a bag of the gentamiacin. The nurse quickly took it to hand it over to the ER doctor.

About an hour later he came back into my room and gave us his assessment. Feeling much relieved to know that he had not done anything wrong, Ed calmed down tremendously. Another doctor came in to review my test results from the x-ray and blood work.

"The damage appears to be isolated to the severe allergic reaction so it looks like you'll not have to be admitted." His words shed much relief on Ed and I both.

The ER doctor came back in explaining that Dr. Anders had immediately changed the antibiotic infusion. A new 3 week supply would be delivered to our home the next day, followed by a visit from the home health nurse. We were to destroy all the gentamiacin. For now, they would get my PICC line started back up, infused, and I could go home. Dr. Anders would run a new series of tests when he removed the PICC line. He would discuss this incident with Dr. Kooper and make sure the lab and test results were faxed to him. In addition, Ed was to call him if there was any medical disruption of any kind.

While I was having the PICC line reinserted Ed called Frannie with the good news. By the time I got home, Frannie came rushing over with her arms full. She had washed and dried my gown already and surprisingly managed to get the blood out. She had chicken soup and club sandwiches. I ate like it was the only talent I possessed. Ed ran over to the nearest Dairy Queen and got us all a banana split while Frannie took control. She greeted the neighbors that stopped by, terrified at the sight of the ambulance at my house again and politely told them I was fine, resting, and she would be sure to tell me they had stopped by.

The next day, another huge box arrived from the medical delivery service and Marilee showed up soon after. She checked me over while Ed counted and signed for the new IV bags of antibiotics. In addition, Marilee had brought some additional prescription items, ordered by Dr. Kooper - vicodin, phenergan and a half dozen epinephrine auto-injectors. Epi pens for allergic emergencies.

To head off Ed's questions, she explained that Dr. Kooper had faxed these orders to Dr. Anders. The nerve damage is having an impact on your immune system. You could easily be allergic to anything, at any time."

"No! Please tell me I won't ever have to go through this again! It was scarier than the aneurysm. I was scared to death, Marilee!"

"That's the reason for the EipPens. So you won't go through it again." She instructed us on how to inject the pen and we moved into the breakfast nook so she could flush my line and refill the infusion with the new antibiotic - just to make sure it was *safe.*

"Are you going to be able to come out every day and do this now. Surely the insurance company knows what happened the last time they insisted I play doctor!"

"I'm afraid I still have orders to come out on Tuesday, Thursday and Saturday."

Ed panicked immediately. "I'm not going to be responsible for killing my wife! You can tell Dr. Anders we'll come into the office. I'll take her to the hospital on Sunday's. This is her life we're talking about! That damn insurance company is not going to risk her life just to save a few dollars!"

After a week indeed, of Marilee, of Dr. Anders nurse and the ER doctor handling the procedure, I got some welcome news. Dr. Anders would remove the PICC line on Wednesday. Test results were great. No more infection. Ed and I both were ready for Wednesday.

Removing it was a lot easier than having it inserted.

I was thrilled so I could only image how Ed felt. No more cumbersome tubing and monitor. No more panic attacks every time Ed came near my left arm. Finally, I was getting better.

I had missed my check up with Dr. Kooper, but with his steady communication with Dr. Stoll and Dr. Anders, he ended up assessing me anyway, from a distance. What's worse, I had missed my CT scan appointment as well as my second session with Dr. Banchly.

Ed and I spent the following weekend talking. I needed to go back to work, desperately. Especially with the promotion and great pay included, it was the only chance we had of getting back into that comfortable, financial position we had once taken for granted.

Ed and I both knew that I was going in the opposite direction, health wise. Especially all these surprises - one after the other. I couldn't grasp enough enthusiasm to propel me back into the work place. Ed decided it was time for him to put in for his retirement. He was well beyond his 30 year tenure, having already hit 35 years with AT&T.

"Your family is the only family I have, too. Let's go ahead and do it - move back to Tennessee. My job was the only thing keeping us here anyway. Just think, you can be near your family. We'll be OK with my pension and selling this house. As soon as you're better, I can find a job there."

I was ecstatic about getting to move back home. We started a list, a long list, of things that had to be done. I had to let Karl know first. That I wouldn't be coming back. Besides, I was due to get another one of those 'Return to work or be fired' letters any day. I perfected my resignation on the computer and mailed it immediately.

The regional boss called. Karl called. They yelled; they begged, and they bribed - a bigger salary, anything I needed, in fact. Even offering to keep the 6 people they had now hired, for me to use as my support staff, for when

I did need to be out of work.

Under normal circumstances, they would have only had to ask once. My mind, however, was still stuck in *sick mode* and magically ignored any sense of work or professional obligations.

In September, Ed and I made the trek to Atlanta, to see Dr. Kooper. Conceding that it probably would be best for me, to be near my family, he would undergo the task to locate and copy my chart for the doctors and specialists in middle Tennessee that were best suited to treat my condition.

No, I wasn't even nearing the recovery stage, especially with all the set backs so far. I've been treated *in moderation,* as that's how all these medical idiosyncrasies have presented themselves. With the sudden and unexpected burning in my right leg, more than likely, the nerve damage was beginning to become a permanent occurrence.

"Since there is no way of knowing what will happen, we can only treat these maladies as they surface. Some may be simple to diagnose and treat; others may be quite difficult. Let's just all hope for the very best. Now, how has the head pain been?"

"It's still there, sometimes really bad and I take a Tramadol and try to sleep. I guess I've just gotten used to it."

"You'll probably have a little bit of pressure for a few more months, maybe even years. As the brain heals, it should start to let up. Of course, for every set back, you almost have to start all over with the healing process."

Promising to call me with the new doctor information, I said a tearful goodbye, hugged him and Ed and I left Dr. Kooper's office for the last time.

Mother and Kathy had been working frantically, looking at houses, and finally found one we could afford on our adjusted income. It was only a mile or so from mother and more important, close enough to my entire family!

It was time for the much delayed CT scan and visit to Dr. Banchly. The hospital and imaging center were only a few blocks apart and the scheduling worked out perfectly. The scan at 9:00 and Dr. Banchly at 11:00.

The scan session was routine, for me anyway. The click, click, rurrrring of the machine penetrated my brain, bringing my thought process to a complete halt. It only took a little over an hour so Ed and I bopped across the street to McDonalds. So I could eat a bite and try to relax for the brain game I still had to endure.

It got off to a great start, with Ed shocked at how fast my brain was letting me spout out the necessary string of words.

Dr. Banchly started with: "Name all the fruits you can, in 60 seconds. Now, vegetables. Good. You're doing great. Most popular surnames; people's last names. Now name all the prominent buildings and monuments you can in 60 seconds."

I was still spouting off answers each time the buzzer rang.

Now the puzzle, I thought wearily, as I was moved over to the large wooden table. Only, this time it wasn't a 9 piece block puzzle.   It was like paper dolls, very light magnetic pieces of clothing and accessories. I had to *dress* the daddy, mommy, little boy and girl.   To complicate it and make it totally impossible for me, there were dozens of non clothing items - hats, caps, purse, briefcase, pipe, necklace, book bag and scarf. I was overwhelmed. It was a total fiasco.

Rather than give up and flunk me, Dr. Banchly pulled another set off the shelf for me to try. A series of buildings for me to place the proper window and doors in. I just sat and stared. It made absolutely no sense whatsoever.

The final try was a world map. Just put each continent and country, ocean and island where they go.   Sure.   I mangled this as well; too many colors for one thing, too many different shapes for another. It's not the world I'm concerned with right now, I argued. It's this horrible, painful pressure inside my head! At this point I couldn't even work a 50 piece jigsaw puzzle.

She was quick to remove my failures from the table before I had a chance to push them off into the floor.

Granted, she gave me twice the allotted time, but I still failed miserably. She walked into the next room and Ed tried, in his own way, to console me. "You've had a rough day; you're just not ready for all this at once. It's O.K. sweetheart."

Dr. Banchly returned with sugar wafers and apple juice. As I sat back to enjoy my refreshments, she and Ed talked.

"I find this hard to believe, Dr. Banchly. At home she can put a 1000 piece puzzle together in one afternoon. You heard the way she spouted out fruits, vegetables and buildings. I probably couldn't name 5 of each. Does she just have an aversion to kindergarten projects?"

"It is fascinating how her mind automatically skips over anything easy or simple. Until I find out otherwise, I can just share with you my preliminary observation. In her mind, she has completed these easy tasks. So quickly that she doesn't even realize it. Her visual receptors know that the correct magnets have already been placed on the family members - in her mind. *That task has already been completed* as far as the actual hand-eye movements are concerned. There is great concern for how fast her mind is moving. It seems to be caused by small bouts of seizure activity, so before I start her on a low dose anti-convulsant, let me confer with Dr. Stoll and Dr. Kooper."

Ed explained our anticipated move to Tennessee and Dr. Banchly quickly agreed to forward copies of my chart to my new therapist, once we were settled and I was medically instructed to go through this again.

By the first day of November, things were coming together in a nice, organized manner. The house was under contract, we had a closing date on our house in Tennessee and were well into the packing stage. I had final visits scheduled with all my other doctors, for a check up and to pick up a copy of my records as well. Dr. Kooper had worked diligently in locating a new team of doctors for me.

We had a quiet, but very nice Thanksgiving dinner with Frannie and Bob. Now less than two weeks before our move, I had worked through all the items on the list, down to the exact day, hour and minute the movers would arrive.

Ed's retirement had been flawless so he was home to help me pretty much of the time, taking over when fatigue forced me to stop and rest. Neither of us could have ever predicted what would happen two nights later.

I woke to a war zone going on in my esophagus, diaphragm, stomach and pancreas. Each organ, fighting to survive, lashing out with horrendous pain. This resulted in another 4 day medical shindig. Endoscopy, colonoscopy, CT scan, bone scan, spinal tap and nerve conduction study.

The lymph nodes in my neck were swollen; the nausea was back and so were the seizures. My esophagus was raw from a constant bout of vomiting. The white blood count in my spinal fluid was elevated. Almost overnight I had developed calcium deposits in my pancreas, lungs and kidneys. More blood clots popped up on my left arm. My potassium level had bottomed out again and on top of all this, the vision in my right eye started fading as my peripheral vision said a final goodbye.

The miraculous workings of the body. In running out of potassium, it instinctively started searching through every cell in my entire body, looking for a hidden supply; just a drop. This was the cause for the majority of pain. With all the vomiting and kidney problems of the past 22 months, the body was no longer able to maintain the proper amount of potassium. Without the intense pain and seizures to alert myself that something was wrong, my lungs would have eventually been paralyzed and even worse, I could have had a heart attack.

"Now, will you put her on a supplement!" Ed demanded, more than asked.

"That would be even more harmful, for her." Dr. Anders asserted. "Her body maintains the right amount of potassium 90 percent of the time. Depletion happens instantly, when she has a vomiting spell or sudden invasion of kidney stones or a seizure, mild or otherwise. Too much potassium would be much worse, and trust me, this is a lot easier to fix, from a medical standpoint. I can give you a list of the warning signs, so you'll know, but I'd definitely get her some medical attention for every vomiting spell. It probably wouldn't hurt to have a weekly blood check."

The nerve conduction test wasn't pleasant by any means, but I'd take that over a spinal tap any day. Lucky me, I had to have both procedures.

Two days later, after another 48 hour date with 'Henry' and the potassium drip, the staff neurologist came in. He had gone over my treatment record and added a new nightmare to his diagnosis.

"The nerve damage from the combination of the aneurysm, hemorrhage and surgery is apparent. You do have peripheral neuropathy, a very painful burning sensation as the nerves short out, throughout the body, with no way to predict when and what part of the body. The damage is irreversible for you, but there are some new medications available to help control it, or at least lessen the pain severity."

"Can you explain this neuropathy, in plain English." Ed asked after seeing my puzzled expression.

Very slowly, the doctor explained, "The neuron cells generate action directives to cells called glial cells which carry out the instructions of the brain. Unfortunately, in your wife's case, so many of the neurons became electrically inactive, dead, and disconnected from the central nervous system. There is no cure, since there's no way to revive dead neuron cells. As the brain sends signals, they skip over the dead neurons, causing intense pain, and pick up instructions again, when they reach living, active neurons. Of course, by then, the instructions have been interrupted and are not complete."

"If it can't be reversed, what does that do to her recovery?"

"This nerve damage is permanent, unfortunately. There is no recovery from it. She will eventually lose the ability to control arm and leg muscles, making mobility very difficult, and in all probability, it will lead to the loss of sensation - to pain, extreme cold, cuts, bruises and general injuries. It can scramble and divert pain sensations, meaning, she may stub her right toe and feel pain in her left thumb."

I was already half asleep as Ed voiced his concerns, frustrations, questions and listened to some more dreadful news.

"The spinal tap helped to relieve most of the white blood count imbalance. She has miniscule stones in both kidneys again, but Dr. Anders wants her to try to flush them out; the reason for the other IV's, in addition to the potassium."

"How long does she have to stay in the hospital this time?"

"Another day at least. I plan on discharging her late tomorrow. Have the nurse page me when you get here to take her home. I know you're moving out of state and I suggest she gets checked out by her new personal physician, internist, neurologist and urologist immediately after you get moved."

"Absolutely. I got the doctor's list from Dr. Kooper already. Believe me, it's my top priority."

I did get to go home the next evening. Ed stopped at the drug store to get my new prescriptions filled, for the burning pain. He came out with 3 bottles of pills. Confused, I started reading the labels. In an instant reflex that came out of the blue, I threw the bottle of phenergan and percocet at him. These aren't doing any good at all, I screamed.

"The doctor prescribed them, so he must think you need them. Let's keep doing what the doctor says, OK?"

"Ed, I'm sick to death of all these pills!"

"I know, sweetheart, but we have to get you well, alright?"

I never did respond, and aptly forgot all about the objection I so readily raised. That night, before supper, I did take a phenergan and finally was able to keep my pimento cheese sandwich and beef stew down.

In between sleeping, taking prescriptions and packing up items we would need in the first few days of our move, I spent hours saying goodbye to friends and neighbors. A week later I was showing significant improvement. The Neurontin seemed to be helping. The movers had come and gone. It was time for us to caravan up I-75. Me, with 800 pages of medical reports and the two boxes of immediate need items; Ed with the computer and printer.

Atlanta morning rush traffic had died down as I drove behind Ed, ever so cautions and alert. I know he was frantic with worry, so close in distance, so far in case of an emergency. My younger brother had eagerly volunteered to fly down and drive me but I was insistent I could make it. Besides, we would be stopping at the exact halfway point - the Cracker Barrel in Dalton.

Part Four

The mind is more powerful than pain
There is no 'h' in sugar
Writing out of necessity
Good day, bad day, great day, sad day
Organized exit, at least

I don't know which of us was more relieved when we pulled into the driveway at my mother's house. Barely had I hugged and kissed her before collapsing in the recliner. Out of pure exhaustion.

Two days later, the movers arrived and we were heavily involved in the unpacking business. I had a slew of family members helping, just to make sure I wouldn't lift, pull or tug anything heavy. Within a week, we were pretty much settled. It was already decided that Christmas would be at my sister Kathy's house and hopefully I could have an extra special Christmas for Ed and I the next year.

We had planned on setting up my initial appointments with the new doctors the week after Christmas. We had to transcend into our new medical pit. My only coverage now was under Ed's retirement plan. Not great, but at least it was something. Our plans were subjected to yet another interruption. The week before Christmas I fell prey to more medical devastation. A month shy of making it two full years. I had two speeds - warp and stop. No middle ground.

The brain seizures were back in addition to the jolts of electricity surging through my right leg.

I liked Dr. Sculley immediately. He had read through my medical records; pages and pages, detailing my ordeal and had me sign forms so he could obtain new test results to compare to my last hospital stay. I was in awe of his quiet, calm demeanor; his intense concern, compassion and determination to help me. I felt greatly relieved to be treated by such a kind, nice and caring doctor.

He reviewed my meds, updated and changed dosages, and encouraged me to see the neurologist right away, explaining that seizures were the result of abnormal brain activity and if left untreated, could cause further damage to the brain. Definitely not good news.

Starting into my third year was bizarre, at best. I had seen my new neurologist and was now back on anti-convulsants. I stuttered instead of speaking; I was impulsive and indecisive, floating through the house, a good 6 inches off the ground at all times. No median. I was a person of extremes, stuck in a perpetual time warp. My mind was quiet for days at a time, and then I would talk for hours straight. At least, I thought I was talking. My words got lost and out of order as they left my brain for that rocket ride out of my mouth. Ed says I created a whole new language, one that only he could understand.

Aluminum foil was now linoleum foil. Googlyoley was really guacamole. In one smooth, overnight transition, I turned to writing. At least, that way, I could go back and correct what I said. I was on my own in the spelling department, though. When I wasn't *writing,* I was studying everything in the house. Making me remember when and where we got each furnishing and memento. Everything else, I questioned - clothes, food, shampoo. All of a sudden, nothing was the right size, color, type or brand.

On a good day, I couldn't get enough done. The entire kitchen had to be cleaned, including the fridge, oven and pantry. That included moving everything off the countertops and washing all the canister sets as well. Food items in the pantry had to be in alphabetical order, by box, can, carton, bag and jar. I would tolerate nothing less.

On a bad day, I didn't know what a kitchen was. I could easily go through a dozen packets of oatmeal trying to fix one serving. Measuring out 2/3 of a cup of water was impossible. I ended up with a bowl full of gooey glob that I couldn't even eat. Cooking was like snow skiing. Looked easy until you got in motion.

What I found impossible to convey to Ed was the simple fact that my brain completed all of these tasks for me. Even produced a visual image of the end result. Telling my hands, 'don't worry about it'. What my hands used to be responsible for doing, my brain now claimed the chore as its very own job duty. That's what I meant all along when I said I was being held captive by my own brain. I just didn't know how to explain it so that someone could understand it. My hands were now fighting my brain over job details and specifics of anything I wanted to do.

I wanted so badly to shine, sparkle or at least have a glimmer of my previous life. Kathy was having a get together dinner and as customary, we all prepared a side dish as she baked, broiled and cooked the main courses. I poured through my recipes and quickly decided that I would make parmesan potatoes. Easy!

At meal time, Kathy and I were both shocked that the

potatoes were barely touched.   Strange, as the whole family was potato eaters. Ed spoke up and said they didn't taste *right*.   I looked at Kathy with fear and she quickly speared one, tasted it quickly and realized the problem.   I had forgotten to boil the potatoes before I sliced them, smothered 'em in butter and parmesan and put them in the oven for 10 minutes. Kathy laughed so I wouldn't be upset at myself and we just made do with the meal sans potatoes.

The seizures? The pills? We didn't know, but I had to start the learning process all over again.   All it took was one quick run through; I caught on pretty fast.   The sad part is that inside my brain, I knew how to cook, tie my shoes, work the can opener and run the dishwasher. I just couldn't get my hands to understand the instructions.

Most days, the floor seemed to have a titled angle to it, making me seem like I was walking sideways around a hillside.   I had to stay in constant motion though, outrunning the burning waves of pain that refused to let go.   For the first few hours after taking my new prescription, Lyrica, the volts of electricity subsided just long enough to plan their next area and intensity of attack. I took full advantage of those few hours; grocery shopping, visiting family, cleaning house and doing some laundry.

Ed had started work at Sanford, on the same night time hours he had just retired from: third shift. He figured it was safer for me to be home at night, so I could sleep and most importantly, he would be at home during the day; in case something happened, in case I had a doctor's visit. He absolutely insisted on going to the doctor with me.

Dr. Sculley had sent me to the hospital for a current set

of film images and new blood work. While waiting for my follow up visit, I moved around the house like a puppet, invisible strings pulling me through each day. Some unknown force guiding me. Then, in an instant, the strings fell down, hanging limp around my feet. Two days before my scheduled appointment, I was catapulted into collapse. Left with a blank mind, frozen stare and explosions of pain.

Another medical surprise! My potassium was all gone, again. Only this time, Ed got me to the hospital before my level dropped too far below the dangerous 2.75 reading. It only took a day and a half to bring it back up enough so my body could function.

No, I still wasn't a candidate for supplements. There was an alternative, though. Along with the gallon of water I was drinking most days, we would add a couple of bananas and one or two slices of apricots. Enough potassium, but not too much.

I was rapidly becoming a nothing person. Stuck in that business acumen of borderline productivity, but which one? Intelligence on ice? Or stupidity on fire? All this knowledge and know-how inside, yet, the thought process deliberately refused to connect. A steadfast partition had formed in my brain, separating the know how from the can do.

I was a human form of Gumby and Pokey. Quick and rambunctious in my mind, slow in the outward follow through. Even my vision was in slow motion, seeing things lopsided and out of proportion. The burning pain got brutal.

It was a constant effort, to try and dig myself out from

this pit my brain had sucked my mind into. I wouldn't have been so insistent, except I knew I was in there somewhere. That proper placement of thoughts, rationale and energetic personality had to come back!

I made it to June before I had another slumber party at the hospital. I was standing at the kitchen sink; Ed beside me fixing a cup of coffee, and he noticed it quickly; before the pain had a chance to attack me. He says my eyes glaze over and just stare straight ahead. Like being in a trance. The pain had just begun when we entered the ER. The seizures started two minutes later.

The minute I woke up and saw the IV drip, I knew what, where and why. Ed came in with a cup of coffee and found me sulking in disgust.

It was Dr. Sculley that actually cheered me up. He was so kind and concerned and as baffled as we were. There was no medical reason for potassium to leave my body so quickly! Unless there was something else going on. Something hidden, that wanted to plan a surprise attack later. Like a spook on Halloween night.

I got to go home the following evening as none of the sequence of tests revealed anything else of potential danger. Ed and I were completely disillusioned. To think there was, for a while, a glimmer of hope.

The entire next month was a nightmare. I couldn't move without screaming in pain. My head was in a vise, the compression was painful. Even the strongest pain pill I had only helped for about 2 hours, knocking me out so I could sleep.

Ed called the neurologist. He reviewed the brain scans.

Nothing new. The midline shift was still prominent, which was certainly a factor. The seizures had removed any effort the brain had made to *settle down*. He had Ed bring me in for a shot of Tegretol. I should have gotten a case of syringes to go. Even though it made me sleep most of the time, it had a tremendous effect on the pain.

I gradually got over the worst of it and withdrew into myself. I was afraid to even open my eyes every morning, fearing what might be in store for me.

I remained closed up in the office all day. Writing. It was a trade off I could live with: bad physical, good mental. Sitting very still in front of the PC, letting my entire life details swirl around in my mind, from age 4 and a watermelon picnic at Ft. Bragg to my first day of school; the exact dress I wore and the Three Musketeers candy bar I had taken for a snack. All the way through my life - I remembered everything. Everyone I had sat by on the hundreds of air flights I had taken for work; school mates, employers, co-workers and business associates. Not only did I recall every person and event, but every word that was ever exchanged.

Because I was hurting so bad, physically, I focused on any and all conversations that had to do with hurt - physical, mental or emotional. A plan was emerging, one that involved my brain and my new thought process. I jumped aboard and started this book.

Three months later, I had a stunning 56,000 words in book format. I was excited at my overall progress. I had finally done something constructive. I called Lou Ellen, a friend of mine; her husband used to write magazine articles for Field and Stream. Telling her about my newfound passion, I asked her opinion and direction. She emailed me a list of a dozen literary agents and attached specific instructions.

Within a month, I had two requests for the entire manuscript! I called Lou Ellen with my explosive news. She talked to Chip, her husband and called me back with his personal view of which agent I should reply to.

After almost 3 weeks, Ms. Naismith actually called. A contract was being drawn up. In the interim, could I possibly increase my word count? For a first novel, it needs to be at least 80,000 to 130,000 words.

Sure, I replied. I'll just dig down in my brain for some more conversations, more details. After all, writing is what I do now. Actually, it's the only thing I *can do* now!

I was relieved for every day that I made it through and fearful of the next day. With the book in editing, proofing and pre-publication, I had months of waiting. The few times I did venture out of the house were when I had a doctor appointment or went Krogering. On rare occasions I did accompany Ed to a couple of his Marine Corps League functions. I enjoyed every outing; every specific event, and especially being around the other Marine wives. The tightly knit bond of true American values was very much apparent. Just being around Dottie, Pam, Betty, Connie, Deanna and Rhonda made me feel so alive! I wanted very much to regain my spirit, to be complete. This group of ladies had a very prominent impact on my struggle to escape from the dark tunnel of desolation I had been in for so long.

I made notes, reminders and lists of things I wanted to

do, needed to do, in hopes of getting better. I spent hours with my best friend, Pat. She had a magical way of pulling out my good parts, making me focus on them, and combat so much of the weariness. We were bonded so tightly that my bad days became her bad days too.

Between the overwhelming kindness and sincerity of the Marine Corps League wives and Pat, I eventually had a mental explosion of optimism. I wanted so badly, to again share their natural display of happiness. For me to do that, I had to concentrate on my condition and learn everything I possibly could about it.

I gathered my copy of the now 800 plus pages of medical notes, records and reports from Acklyn. I read through pamphlets and brochures that Stella had brought to me during my year of home health visits. Though interesting, not one of them gave me information that would help me. Everything was simply a review of the brain, and things that can happen to the brain. Nothing about what happens to you once something happens to the brain.

That's when I decided to write this book. Not only for me, recounting and confronting my ordeal, but for so many others, devoid of understanding, of knowing what might and could happen during the recovery process. I called and wrote and emailed every doctor I had seen in any capacity, since the aneurysm. I was startled at the response from some, as well as the lack of it from others.

With my brain now content with my lack of adventure and extroverted excitement, I became solely focused on this project.

For me, it seemed that seclusion was my survival. My world of daily pain kept reminding me, *my clock is ticking.* I had to write this book. So that others who find themselves in a world of the unknown after a ruptured aneurysm would perhaps find their strengths and capabilities as well. Keep turning over the rocks until something jumps out. It took me over 2 years.

My neurologist says I fought so hard to find my real self that I sort of outsmarted the damages and burst out with this latent career before the brain realized what was happening. I had the inner strength to realize that the mind is more powerful than pain. Thank goodness for that positive aspect.

I seem O.K. as long as I focus every ounce of intensity on one thing at a time and just one thing.

I researched every major neurological center in the U.S., calling, writing and emailing. I was literally stunned at the overwhelming amount of assistance I was receiving, especially from two of the largest and most prominent medical facilities - Cedars-Sinai and the National Institute of Health. Along with the half dozen or so doctors that assisted me, I was suddenly surrounded by a world of medical expertise.

As I read each report, summary and translation of my actual records, I was keenly aware of the powerhouse of knowledge I had accumulated. Yet, none of it was good news. I did, at least have a more thorough understanding of what had happened to me.

The medical world doesn't have a step-by-step guide for ruptured brain aneurysm survival. Because each person's brain is a one-of-a-kind schematic, unique to their own exclusive being. Survival stands at an infinitesimal number. I'm left in the dark as to what bridges there are left to cross.

My brain continues its series of somersaults; one day probing me to concentrate and to function. The next day, refusing to give me any sign of normality. I have come to recognize those days, as they're always preceded by the click, click, click sound during the night. The sound of my own skull, shifting, trying to piece itself back together, searching for the missing bone particles so it can be whole once again.

Outside, the world was going on around me. I didn't care, simply because I didn't know how to care. As long as I sat perfectly still, moving only my hands, as I keyed, I was relieved of pain. It became my life, in most ways. Until Thanksgiving. No way was I going to miss dinner at Kathy's. Being around my family gave me a warm sense of contentment; an emotional treasure of sorts.

I turned away from writing long enough for Ed to take me on a couple of Christmas shopping excursions, decorate the house for the holidays and put up the tree.

Our wedding anniversary was December 10th. I gave in to Ed's pleas to at least go out to eat. Fearing that a long ride would invoke another spell of nausea, we selected a nearby restaurant. A new one, in fact - Ruby Tuesday's. All dressed up and ready to dine.

As soon as Ed parked the car, the pain hit like a rocket propelled firestorm. Something was definitely being roused from a state of hibernation. I bit my fingers, lips and tongue to keep from crying out and ruining our dinner. When Ed came around to open the car door for me, he immediately saw that something wasn't right.

"I'm O.K. It's O.K." I insisted. "It's nothing. Just a little discomfort. It'll pass." I assured him.

We got seated pretty quickly for a Saturday night. With the menu open in front of me, the vivid laminate pictures of food began swirling around; the wording was smudges I couldn't begin to read. Intent not to ruin our night, I pointed to an image when the waitress arrived to take our order. Beef tips, I heard Ed say.

He kept asking if I was O.K. I kept muttering uuuhhh, huhhhhh. Until I could bear it no longer and the rivets of pain soared through me with the speed of an F11 fighter jet. I started fading into a world I had known so many times before – near blackness; the edge of nothingness.

Ed yelled for the waitress, told her to pack our food to go and started helping me on with my coat. Seeing our predicament, she offered to call for an ambulance.

"No." I mumbled. "I'm O.K."

"Let me get her to the car and I'll be right back." Ed quickly stated.

By the time he got me to the exit, the waitress came running up with a brown carry bag. Ed set me down in the waiting area booth, counted out some money and ran back over to me. By the time we got to the hospital, I was screaming in pain, unable to stop the stream of tears caused by my agony. Once inside, I staggered to the most remote section of the waiting room and collapsed, hoping I was far enough away from the whispers and stares my moaning would generate.

Ed signed me in, sat next to me and tried to comfort me while we waited. It was less than 5 minutes later, Ed said, that a male nurse came scurrying down the hall with a wheelchair. My pain kept me from realizing that this was a familiar being.

The same ER doctor who had so precisely and wonderfully handled so many of my medical emergencies before.   Ed filled him in on my sudden barrage of symptoms enroute to triage.

Having such a vivid remembrance of my situation, the first thing was pain management, so I could endure the batch of tests that would follow.

Out of the blue, once again, my body was depleted of potassium. In addition, my CT scan showed an anomaly in my kidney.

On the positive side, I was being treated by two of the best ER doctors; ones I felt so comfortable around, accustomed to their sincere and expert care. Dr. Sculley was contacted as I was being admitted, confined once again, by 'Henry', the IV pole.

Ed knew I was sick, not only physically, but because I had ruined our anniversary. He tried to make light of it, cheer me up, by jokingly asking, "Just think, how many other couples do you think have spent their anniversary in the hospital?"

We knew I would be stuck, from two to four days, depending on how low my potassium level had dropped, and how long it would take for my blood pressure to stabilize.

The pain infusion, doing its job of controlling the roaring furnace inside me, extended its side effect, making me sleep.

Ed arrived early the next morning, as I was working on the 7:00 breakfast tray. He talked with the staff at the nurse's station while I was helped with the bathing and dressing ritual.

Right before 8:00, both Ed and I were graced with a most welcome site. Dr. Sculley had no doubt disrupted his entire Sunday schedule, because of me. I felt horrible and began apologizing. He wasn't concerned about his weekend. He was concerned about me. I know that if it was medically, or humanly possible, he would have vanquished my pain on the spot. He's very compassionate and caring that way.

The most pressing issue was to restore an adequate amount of potassium to my body, get my blood pressure back to normal, make sure this incident didn't invoke a series of seizures and then get my kidney problem resolved.

He had called my urologist; I had to get medical treatment as soon as I was able; as soon as possible.

Dr. Sculley left to check on the results from my 6:00 A.M. blood work. Ed and I just looked at each other. There was nothing to say. We had been through this so much we knew it was a standard time frame with no way out.

It was making me crazy, going for weeks, even months, with the head pain and neuropathy only. My whole life, every facet, had changed so dramatically, but I had slowly adjusted. With Ed's help, we had targeted the specific changes and I learned to live with them.

I could no longer talk while in motion. I had to be sitting or standing. I couldn't do both. It was either talk or walk. One or the other.

I had grown accustomed to life going on around me, helpless to be a part of it. I could only watch, hypnotized by the thick layer of foggy cushioning in my brain.

There would be no more multi-tasking for me. No chatting away on the phone as I cooked. No ironing and watching CNN at the same time.

Ed and I were both terrified. I had made it through only half of the predicted 5 years I was given. Every time we thought I had reached a level stage, where I would remain until I got better, I was launched backwards.

The one thing that remained a constant, viable, undangered area was my mind. It seemed to be the only thing that steered clear from these physical explosions.

I convinced Ed to go eat when my lunch tray arrived. I called mother and Kathy, assuring them I was fine, just resting mostly. I would be going home practically any time, I insisted, to keep them from visiting. I couldn't bear for anyone to see me in this helpless state. If by chance, I didn't get to go home, yes, I would let them know and they would happily bring me some goodies - books, magazines, candy, gum, or anything my heart desired.

Ed returned as the nurse was taking my vitals and checking the IV. The pain med was keeping me drowsy.

It was about 2:00 when Dr. Tilton came strolling in, with his natural style and charm, a distinct credit to the entire urological profession.

"Oh no!" I gasped. "I've upset your Sunday also."

"That's O.K. I had a consultation over here anyway. I would have come to check on you regardless. Don't give it another thought."

That relieved me greatly and he told us that he had talked to Dr. Sculley and had stopped by radiology to pick up my report. "You have stones in both kidneys, again. The right one shows stones that are small enough for you to hopefully pass."

"The left kidney warrants enough concern that I need another scan - a contrast scan. It's quite enlarged and I don't see any way around surgery. As soon as you are discharged, I want you to go straight to Heartfield for a scan. Bring the images, which they'll put on disk for you, straight to my office so we can discuss our surgical options."

"Now, let me go check on your potassium level. If it has improved significantly, Dr. Sculley and I already agreed that I would discharge you. If that's the case, I want you at Heartfield tomorrow, and I'll see you after the scan."

Dr. Tilton left and the tears started flowing. I couldn't make it 6 months without a hospital stay or surgery. This was devastating. I was overwhelmed with all the confusion. How could my mind be so strong and my body be so weak? For a while, I was content with being half a person. Now, I was much less than half. Ed tried, but I was inconsolable, frantic with worry that I couldn't possibly survive much longer.

My fiction book was due to roll off the press at any time and my agent was furious. I had missed countless conference calls, emails and phone calls. I absolutely refused to let her know I was a physical disaster. I would get better; I insisted on nothing less. I had a sequel planned and most important of all, I had this book.

Dr. Tilton did get me discharged late that evening. Only so I could go home, sleep, get up and get ready for another medical outing.

Another lithotripsy procedure, Dr. Tilton had said.

The left kidney was twice the normal size, swollen again because of a large, 5 centimeter stone, almost 2 inches in size! I could rest for one day and undergo the procedure on the following morning.

It was pretty routine for Dr. Tilton, I'm sure, but for me, it was just as routine. Later that afternoon, Ed got me home and started forcing the pain pills and antibiotics down me. The soreness and bruising, I knew would go away in a few days. I didn't expect the added complications though.

Dr. Tilton stressed that he was pleased with my relatively quick recovery and then very carefully and slowly informed me that not only was my body unable to maintain a normal amount of potassium, but now I was zero, zip, completely out of the 3 major hormones - testosterone, estrogen and progesterone. The hormone depletion was affecting my whole system. Corticosteroid production was vital to the body. It was a job usually carried out by a natural supply of progesterone. My body now lacked the tools to perform this task. Without a balance of these three hormones, I was well set up for easy bone fractures.

The remedy? I had to take hormone therapy to a whole new level. A pill would do more damage than good, considering the state of my kidneys. I had to have a special compound made just for me by a pharmacal chemist. So I could feed it onto my wrist daily, by way of a medicine dropper.

My follow up visit with Dr. Sculley was just as dismal. From all the frantic worry, disgust and frustration, I now had an extremely ulcerated stomach, swollen lymph nodes and inflamed esophagus. Other organs were protesting as well - diaphragm, pancreas and intestines - no doubt from the brain directive for my body to perform a desperate, thorough search for potassium.

Lucky for me, both the colonoscopy and endoscopy were carried out during the same OR scheduling. The damage was repairable, however, with a daily regimen of pills, lots of pills.

Latent damage. Complications. Three years later. The body functioning brain impulses weren't getting through. The nerves were too severely damaged, like wires stripped of their insulation; naked and useless. I was a V8 engine now hitting on just 4 cylinders.

The brain was refusing to heal; balking over the midline shift; not liking its new crooked environment. It wanted what it had been used to for so many years - a nice symmetrical position.

It was spring time before I gathered my remaining resources and got back to my writing project. Hating every pill I had to swallow; but hating the pain even worse. The zaps of electricity in my leg were getting more severe, making sleep impossible. I grew very adapt at working fiendishly for the two hours following my seizure pills. That was the only time pain diminished enough to let me think.

When the rare appearance of a hunger sensation did surface, it seemed like nothing in the kitchen appeared appetizing so Ed rushed me to Kroger's and patiently waited while I searched the aisles, looking for something that piqued my appetite.

I located my doctor ordered low sodium foods in the Lean Cousine section, and honestly couldn't resist Boston Market's Spinach and Artichoke dip. Hey, it's a start, I told Ed.

And, for a few, wonderful days, I was superwoman again. Flying through the house, happily giving in to the demands of all chores, even squeezing in a delightful visit with Pat. Maybe all the pills had finally forced my brain to relax, to shut up and be still.

I was back in the good graces of my agent, as we talked and made publishing plans for this book and my fiction sequel. Yes, I had decided on a pen name for my fiction works, I told Andrea - June Gavin. June, for my birth month. Gavin, for Hollywood's own John Gavin. My screen idol, ever since I watched *Backstreet* and *Imitation of Life*, still two of my most favorite movies.

The month of June found me back in the hospital again. By now, I was definitely on a first name basis with the ER doctors. What Ed and I assumed was another potassium depletion turned out to be something very different. Fibroid cysts. Hundreds of them. Thanks to the lack of hormones, this was the retaliation. With the daily compound drops, my body had not yet had time to build up a sufficient volume. From my neck to my waist. You could map it out in one inch squares. Draw a dot inside each one. That's where I hurt. To touch any of the dots caused immense pain. It was like having 100 toothaches all at once, all over your body.

A pain injection and more narcotics was the only treatment. I spent the next three weeks huddled up in the corner of the sofa. Afraid to move because I couldn't tolerate the pain. The pills were so strong I stayed nauseated. Ed had to start cutting them in half again.

I begged Dr. Sculley to cut them out. All of them. Just take your scalpel and get these cysts out of me! I was very serious. He educated me by explaining that the scar tissue would be much worse. He made his point.

I had no choice but to endure it; wait it out. Until my body had stored an adequate amount of the hormone compound. As that volume in my body increased, the inflammation will begin to subside. May take two months, maybe six, I was told. It took exactly 4 months.

As I huddled on the sofa, a pillow over my stomach for protection, I read through the medical data. I was receiving batches daily, by mail and email. I printed everything out and carefully unfolded the postal offerings, carried everything into the den and read for hours. For no apparent reason, I would start crying, or laughing, or talking about an article I had read months ago. Ed says my brain was like a square peg; it no longer fit in the round hole. More like Humpty Dumpty, I told him. I couldn't be put back together either.

The cyst inflammation began decreasing. The nerve pain was taking on a personality of its own. What's worse, it moved in and planned to stay.

During my cyst check-up, Dr. Sculley became quite concerned about the relentless nerve pain and immediately arranged for me to have a current nerve conduction study. Dr. Estes, the neurologist that conducted this test, was so concerned about my new 10 pound weight loss and the lack of response I was getting from the anti-convulsants that he sent me to an associate, a neurological pain specialist, for his professional assessment.

That assessment led to a sleep study, especially since Ed was so gracious in responding to his question about how much sleep I was getting; approximately 3 hours a night and 3 or 4 ten minute naps per day.

Sure enough, the findings were horrible. Two sessions resulted in like findings. I woke up 87 times the first night and 117 times the second night; every time the electrical volts surged through my abdomen and down my leg.

The only escape was more drugs. Strong enough to be called dreamland drugs. Anti-convulsants so strong they forced my brain to rest. I had to admit, though, my sleep did increase to an astonishing 5 hours a night. They sure messed up my attempts to walk more than a few feet at a time though.

I turned my attention to anything that required intense, steady thought. Anything to escape the pain. I worked a dozen complicated jigsaw puzzles and then started keying everything in sight. I keyed lists. Lots of lists. I keyed a list of the title of every CD and DVD music and movie disk I had in the house. Every book, by title and then by author.

My brain had rotated. The more complicated the task, the more I felt human. I became obsessed with my computer. I dissected the hard drive, recouping every document and image I had ever installed, downloaded, viewed or received via email. I sorted and grouped and filed and deleted until I was content my hard drive was now in order.

Then, I started keying in recipes, mostly in an attempt to get them all in one place, in one neat file. Once finished, I printed them all out to bind in one 3 ring binder. First, I had to separate them: main dishes, meat dishes, casseroles, breads, salads and desserts. As I sorted, I saw a mis-type, and then another one, and another. My whole project, half ruined. Hopefully it affected only the desserts, as I read through each one.

They would all have to be fixed, and re-printed. On every single one, I had keyed sugar as 'shugar'. I was exasperated as I went back into the word processor to fix them all, reprint them and then bind them.

When I finished with that project, I turned to something slightly different. Still intent to concentrate, though, I must have gone through 300 Qtips and 2 whole bottles of alcohol when I decided all the heat and air vents in the house needed to be cleaned. Ed woke up to get ready for work just as I was finishing up.

After I answered his question as to what was I doing, he casually pointed out that the vents easily 'lift out'. Telling me wasn't enough; he had to show me how very easy it was to lift them out of the floor. Wouldn't it have been much easier to wash them in the sink, he asked.

"Well, yes. I wanted to clean them this way." I quickly added. There was no way I was going to admit that *I didn't think* of the easy way.

My head pain had reached a new degree of hurt by the end of July. Ed rushed me to Dr. Sculley. Thank heavens he wasn't too busy this particular morning. I stepped up and sat on the exam table and he began his routine - temperature, blood pressure, eyes, nose, mouth and ears, for starters. He stopped suddenly and asked how long my ear had been hurting.

"My ear?"

"You have a serious ear infection. It has to hurt. That's part of the peripheral neuropathy; loss of pain sensation. Let's get you on some antibiotics, quickly. I'll go ahead and give you an injection, in case you do start to feel it hurting."

"Does that affect her head pain, make it worse?" Ed asked.

"It could have some effect, but I wouldn't rule out a little bit of sinus infection either. To be on the safe side, let's go ahead and see an ENT doctor."

Luckily, Kathy got me an appointment with Dr. Crestley the same week. No, it wasn't a sinus infection. Allergies. Tons of them. To every thing in the universe. Some just in the beginning stages; some severely. Shots wouldn't even help.

I was devastated, again. Frantic with the realization that this might just be as good as it's going to get for me. I worked myself into a frenzy, and had my heart pounding right out of my chest, hurting and pinching.

After a consultation with the most wonderful cardiologist, and considering my degraded state, fearing there might be some nerve damage going on that was now affecting my heart, Dr. Branson put me through the entire litany of tests. My heart was fine. The neuropathy was the big worry, the culprit of all my problems.

I was sent to Nashville, to the neurological division at the Neurological Center. Dr. Grayson studied my films from the past 3 years, did a thorough exam and ultimately concurred - the neuropathy had taken firm root. It was now as much a part of me as my own skin.

That was hard enough to hear, but even worse was hearing that the head pain was justified. A slow and steady series of seizures had begun. Treatment was urgent, as these seizures meant the gradual destruction of brain cells.

The fortunate part, there was a new, highly effective medication that would hopefully help me. If, however, it generated no significant relief, there were a couple of new treatments I could undergo.

Ed and I listened intently as he summarized: I had the most lingering, debilitating, irreversible complication that a ruptured aneurysm and subarachnoid hemorrhage could cause. The network of nerves that transmit information from the central nervous system to every part of the body has been damaged. The pain is excruciating, and probably, he said, if all my pain sensors were working, I'd be screaming.

Peripheral neuropathy basically distorts and interrupts messages between the brain and the rest of the body. Making you unable to register normal sensations. The nerve fibers most distant from the brain usually malfunction first.

The electrified pain sensations will spread, usually causing organ failure. Again, in my case, there is no cure. Surgery to repair nerve damage is normally effective in cases where the nerve has only been compressed. Mine had been severed, cauterized, clipped and destroyed.

Diminishing the pain and slowing the damage rate is the immediate treatment plan. Then, we'll go from there after the first of the year, the doctor told me.

It would be so very easy to succumb to this pain, let it swallow me into an endless realm of nothingness, but some invisible strength keeps forcing me to charge ahead; keep trying to outrun the pain, endure it and outlast it.

With the help of Trilepital, I was able to climb out of the pain pit, somewhat. I wrote, sewed, cooked and cleaned. For every really great day I had, it was followed by one or two really bad days, but I figured the trade off was worth it. Just to have a good day.

In the very depths of my thoughts, I was determined not to give in. Complaining, or even acknowledging any pain would surely send me right back to the hospital and that triggered no general excitement.

I prayed that I would be able to just accept pain and live without benefit of thriving; just existing and accomplishing what little I could.

On most days, the Trilepital was helping. Allergies kept my throat inflamed and swollen, so Ed and I put several air purifiers throughout the house. I was on a mission of a different sort, each day trying to find foods that didn't propel too much of a reaction. A daily series of trial and error. Bread was fast becoming a major culprit, followed by bananas. My list of 'can't eats' was rapidly growing. It seemed like the only safe foods so far were vegetables, candy and cantaloupe.

The constant fear of something else going wrong or running out of potassium again kept me now both mentally and physically bogged down.

I zoom through good days with no apparent sign of damage, minimal mobility problems, mastering incredible feats. On one really good day, I can easily key 4000 words to my sequel or write 3 dozen strings of commands for my inventory program I'm creating, so that I can neatly categorize everything in the house; by room, and still manage basic household duties.

It frightens me that I have no control over these messages my brain is sending out; the commands for me to be organized to the point of obsessing about it. My brain *makes me* rush through a series of tasks and I'm not even sure why! Every bottle of nail polish has to be lined up on the shelf, according to height and shape of the bottle. Every pair of shoes has to be in its own plastic bin, *and labeled* as to color, brand and season! I just follow the commands..... I have to get organized!

Then, without warning, my brain takes a break; shuts down; goes on vacation. These are very difficult days. I have no *directions.* I'm alone with the slow sizzle of seizures and burning legs. These are bad days for me, but they're really bad for Ed. I can't make a complete sentence and writing is all but legible. I still make notes and lots of lists. Want lists, wish lists, need lists and grocery lists.

Ed finally confronted me about my writing, which used to be so neat, so delicate and easy to read. Handing me a note I had written on a *bad day,* I took it and stared at it, concentrating with all my might. I couldn't understand what he was trying to tell me!

"Look at it, sweetheart! It's backwards! Every word is written backwards! I have to hold it up to the mirror to read it!"

Oops. I still didn't understand what was wrong. He grabbed a handful of notes and reminders from the desk tray. They were all in my new writing style. What really freaked him was how quickly and precisely I read them, without a mirror.

"That's not even the bad part. Look at this! Is this a grocery list?"

I read the list and even I could see the problem with this. Even though it wasn't written backwards, it was a nightmare to interpret: s/mete, cheze, spunges, butr, shugr, razens, pars.

"Well, if I was going to the store with this list, I'd get sandwich meat, cheese, sponges, butter, sugar, raisens and pears. My mind just moves faster than my writing hand does."

"You go back to the eye doctor next month. We'll be sure to ask him what's causing this. Something in your eyes is definitely misaligned. I have no doubt that every string of text, every word in your mind, is meticulously formed and spelled. But, by the time it fruit loops through the damaged nerves, it comes out in a broken mess."

His words stung so bad I'm making a really strong effort not to write anything by hand.

He came in from work one morning and told me he found a dead bird beside the garage access door. Probably flew into the door glass, he said.

"Well, you fly or you die" was my only remark. I never even formatted the words; they just fell out. How do you make someone understand you aren't really saying what they hear you say?

Ed calls it reverse intelligence. I call it instant stupidity, recalling one bright Friday morning that mother and I had an outing planned. As was the routine, I made the short one mile drive over to her house and she drove from there. I showered and dressed, excited about feeling well enough to get out of the house. I got to mothers, parked the car and bopped up the steps where she was holding the door open. We hugged and kissed and she suddenly exclaimed, "Do you know you have your house shoes on?"

Looking down, I gasped in horror. Yes, I had managed to get ready, grab purse and car keys; never giving a thought to my shoes. I ended up wearing a pair of hers; one size too large, but I managed.

By the beginning of fall, I was in a clearly justified state of anxiety. My first book was published and I was right in the middle of reviews, interviews, the cover design for this book and wrapping up the sequel.

I refused to even think about my ticking clock; that things could change in an instant. I gave up even trying to explain to Ed how I felt, when I had a bad day. I couldn't even explain it to myself. How do you intelligently explain that your brain feels like a glob of Jell-O. Slamming against the side of your skull every time you move your head. And my leg, feeling as if it's constantly being zapped with a stun gun.

I had a follow up with my nerveologist, as Ed called him. For another nerve conduction test; acupuncture of the leg, it seemed like. Dr. Estes reassured me that he felt the Trilepital was helping, giving me as much relief as I could get, until Dr. Grayson could determine the next treatment plan.

"Every attempt your brain makes to *settle down* redefines your entire being. Every time the brain shifts, trying to compensate for the uneven position, it reorganizes your thought process. This could be a daily, weekly or monthly event. Your personality constantly changes - from serious to hilarious, introvert to extrovert, thorough to haphazard. You can't pinpoint specific pain - kidney stones never hurt, ear infections don't exhibit the slightest hint of pain, yet, paper cuts hurt tremendously. You seem to experience the most pain when your potassium level drops. Your brain knows it is out of alignment and it keeps trying to reposition itself. It resents, tremendously, the fact that your brain cavity has been altered, changing the normal path your brain waves traveled for so many years."

To compensate for my bad days, I picked up even more speed on my good days, moving quickly from task to task. I spent hours on the phone, talking to family and friends. I flew through housework, paid bills on line, updated and managed my web site, worked on my inventory program, researched trivia items I wanted to know more about, breezed through conference calls with my agent and publisher and talked to other authors.

I moved so fast that I didn't have time to listen to what my brain was telling me. I was obsessed with cramming 40 hours into one good day.

On a bad day, there is no escape. I can't generate my own thoughts. They're formed without my input or consent. The intensity of the danger message frightens me, but it's far too late. I'm already obsessed, with organization. I am a stranger to myself. Personifying someone I don't know at all; a person of extremes. Talking constantly for hours, blunt to the point of shock. And, then, at other times, you couldn't force conversation from me at gunpoint.

The body is dying while the mind lives on. At least that's how I feel on a bad day. I still search my mind, for an answer, a miraculous, logical way out of this physical mess. That's how I happened upon the startling revelation; that's how I learned about death. The entire 10 days I was in a state of unconscious darkness in NICU, I could have just as easily been dead. That's the thing about death I figured out.

When you die, you don't know you're dead. You don't

know anything. There exists no longer a concept of life. You just drift off and swoosh into an eternal whisp of air, where I was for those 10 days. On a good day I realize that survival is a treasure, and I'm thankful for every minute. I continue to pray for all aneurysm survivors, that we may improve, and in due course, recover.

I sincerely hope this book provides some source of understanding; that a ruptured aneurysm has tragically dented us, hasn't totally destroyed us, but the changes we are forced to go through are so complex. For this reason, I know the price is high. I wrote this book for us and for our families. So that they may understand that, on our bad days, we are still there. Submerged under the layers of damage, but still possessing every human value, degree of determination, intellect and sense of kindness that we've always had.

I know that I've lost some sense of mobility, sight, sensation and most of the normal, happy aspects of life. Just as I know that I've gained, or found - a lot of skills I didn't have access to before: programming, writing, fierce attention to details, concentration and organizational skills. I know my kidneys are distressed and my immune system is shot.

I have no peripheral vision and still have seizures. I can't do just *anything* and my potassium level will always be borderline. I fully realize the peripheral neuropathy is worsening.

Most of all, I know, *I have to believe* that my mind is the most powerful thing about me right now. It has to remain strong – stronger than the pain.

When I began this book I had no idea how extremely difficult it would be to tell my story. But, after talking with a few other survivors, I easily realized that I was telling their story also.

The hard part was realizing that a good day can quickly turn into a bad day.

The easy part of writing this book was recalling that Saturday morning in January when my head exploded.

The End

Cedars-Sinai Medical Center

The Maxine Dunitz Neurological Institute is dedicated to advancing the field of neurosurgery, offering a full spectrum of treatment options and developing promising protocols for neurological diseases that are extremely difficult to treat with conventional therapies.

Under the direction of Keith L. Black, M.D., institute neurosurgeons and neuro-oncologists treat the full range of conditions affecting the brain, spinal cord and nerves. Because no two individuals respond in the same way to treatment, the multidisciplinary team of specialists provide highly individualized diagnostic and treatment services.

You can visit Cedars-Sinai Medical Center on line:

www.csmc.edu

National Institute of Neurological Disorders & Stroke (NINDS) located in Bethesda, Maryland, NINDS was created by the U.S. Congress in 1950 and is one of more than two dozen research institutes and centers that comprise the National Institute of Health. It is an agency of the Public Health Service within the U.S. Department of Health and Human Services. NINDS has occupied a central position in the world of neuroscience for over 50 years.

Astoundingly, more than 600 disorders afflict the nervous system, which brings us to the mission of the NINDS - to reduce the burden of neurological disease, a burden affecting every age group and segment of society throughout the world. The Institute funds research training and development to help build the next generation of neuroscientists as well as serving as a prime source of neurological information for scientists, clinicians and the public.

Alan P. Koretsky, Ph.D., is the Scientific Director of NINDS. Under his direction is the NINDS division of Intramural Research, conducting studies on the biomedical processes involved in more than 600 disorders and conditions that affect the nervous system.

National Institute of Health
www.nih.gov

National Institute of Neurological Disorders and Stroke
www.ninds.nih.gov

Author's Summation~

Basic knowledge lets us realize that, like a snowflake or DNA profile, everyone has a distinctly different brain schematic, as witnessed by our character, mannerisms, verbiage style, demeanor, compassion, faith and even sometimes, malice.

For the majority of us, we are kind, educated, experienced and laden with only the best combination of moral integrity and benevolence, graciously exhibiting our personality traits to family and friends, work peers, community and business associates and quite frequently, the general public.

Imagine waking up one morning and not being able to exhibit any portion of yourself. In a matter of seconds during the night, the entire structure of your character had vanished; ceased to exist. That is exactly what happened to me on January 25, 2003.

As human beings, our brains are distinct in the sense that directives are issued via the thought process, throughout the 30,000 nerve cells and 100 billion neurons within the central nervous system.

Like a quarterback handing off the football, these directives are passed along to neurons in the expedient, direct and habitual sequence that defines our character. If a verbal response is necessary, the brain will search until it finds the correct group of words for the proper reply. If an action is required, the brain sends the correct signal – whether instructing you to shake hands, sit down or scratch an itch.

After a ruptured aneurysm, these signals become pooled

together, overlapping and criss crossing, no longer able to act independently in the normal and proficient manner they had always been accustomed to.

Directives now rush to the neurons in a haphazard manner, confused by the unwelcome intrusion that the damage and surgery caused. Every trait that you ever possessed is still there, but because of the trauma, you are now a stranger to the message sending center of your own brain. It no longer knows that you pour milk on your oatmeal, that you possess a marvelous talent for painting, that you have a passion for hunting or that you've always enjoyed gardening. It is now a pretty useless computer, stripped of its programming.

It's not that you have a memory problem. The damage has simply scattered and buried these aspects of your life all throughout your brain, in a most unorganized fashion. Propelling the most important facets of your character to the most remote sections of your remaining gray matter, replacing the daily tasks, enjoyments and responsibilities with things of little importance.

Perhaps you've never had a real fondness for classical music but you find it is suddenly very enjoyable. You've never really had any desire for seafood and now you want to dine at Red Lobster, Joe's Crab Shack, Captain D's or the New Orleans Manor every chance you get.

You suddenly despise coconut and roast beef, two of your favorite foods, at least, they were *before the aneurysm.*

You used to enjoy a healthy variety of social entertainment, whether it was going to the movies, dining out or attending a family gathering. You now fear any social event, overwhelmed at the potential of crowds, the swirling mass of activity.

The brain reprogramming takes a very long time and an awful lot of determination – to locate those characteristics that were once so vital to your very being.

You've always prided yourself on being objective, able to see both sides of issue, regardless of its importance in your life. You now find yourself somewhat biased and firm in your opinions. Personal views are difficult to understand and rationalize. You play a constant game with your mind – a competition of sorts, trying in earnest to force it to return to normal. Restore you to the original person you were for so many years. Bring back your original ways and methods that you felt comfortable with. You are suddenly a stranger to yourself, and even worse, you are helpless to initiate any improvement.

Your expensive Anne Klein and Perry Ellis suits used to fit so well, and you truly were comfortable in your casual attire of Members Only, Hilfiger, Bobbie Brooks and Dockers. They now seem as strange and useless as wasabi sauce. Appearance used to be everything, a task you accomplished with natural ease, without any difficulty. It's now impossible to understand the importance or reason to be personally and professionally well dressed. You can no longer coordinate outfits; that talent is long gone.

You've played tennis once a week for most of your adult life and you suddenly wake up one day, unable to even make it to the court, much less play the game. You're only vaguely aware through bits and pieces of visual images that you ever played tennis at all.

Even walking is a difficult, cumbersome task. You can no longer carry on a conversation as you walk. Your mind is busy, constantly reminding you to put one foot in front of the other. A curb, step or missing chunk of walkway is a disaster. Instructions from the brain are no longer instantaneous. You have to search for each and every one. There are no more simultaneous messages to coordinate actions. Each movement is a separate task.

The same mass of instruction generators in your brain; the ones that tell you when to talk, quickly search your memory bank for a particular person's name, provide an accurate response to a question or simple driving directions to your own house are the very same group of cells that instruct your body how to function. The systematic and orderly process of vital organ function and explicit control of your extremities has now been infringed up. There are no more divider lines on your internal road system.

It can medically be referred to as fortunate, that you didn't lose your entire ability to see, speak or walk. Unfortunately, you lost a portion of each. Like a prized figurine that has been dropped and broken. All the major pieces are there, but the damage has been done. Even an attempt to glue it back together will not restore it completely.

With craniotomy surgery for a ruptured aneurysm, dozens of nerves in the brain are destroyed, severed by the artery bursting and taking many with it, in the explosion. Many are clipped and demolished during the surgery itself, in order to get to the site of the rupture. The dissected ends aren't reattached. They remain separated, each end cauterized, forever ending that connection, once so vital in transporting instructional directions throughout your body.

Part of your brain matter is lost as well, damaged by the hemorrhage after the rupture. Each second the brain is surrounded by the pooling blood and incredible pressure, brain tissue is destroyed, obliterating all parts of your character and memory that it once housed. The brain retaliates, not accepting the now empty portion inside your head, where active, living tissue once rested. It is forced to shift its position and in the process, voice its adamant dislike with an ongoing series of seizures. Meanwhile, the four groups of nerves branching from the spinal cord realize they have been damaged as well, and begin sending sporadic volts of electrified pain throughout your body.

In my case, the signals that tell me what hunger means, the distinction between sadness and laughter, the instruction for my cells to store and release potassium in a normal manner have all been terminated. The damage was far too much for the body to compensate for. There is no reserve supply of neurons.

The brain, however, complete with its own strange and unique backup system tries to make amends as best it can. It continues to send signals despite the fact that they've got nowhere to go. Signals dedicated to the daily operation of abilities you no longer have. As with me, the ability to feel specific types of pain as well as the inability to feel normal pain were right in the midst of damages. A normal pain, such as toothache or earache goes completely unnoticed while the intensity of pain from the smallest bruise can send me into an unbearable state of distress.

Survival itself isn't simply the aspect that you are still

alive. It encompasses a host of facets. Survival is much more than physical endurance and coping with pain. It is the tolerance of a forced, strange and unknown way of life that arrives during recovery. It sadly encompasses the ability to defeat so many obstacles – physical, emotional, financial and professional. Without recouping these four elements of life, there is no survival; just the stark realization that you're still in a semi-recovered state.

I know, because I still remain in the depths of recovery, struggling every day to accomplish some act of constructive prominence. My spoken words, most often, continue to display a clear indication of damage. Walking at a faster pace than baby steps is usually a physical disaster. Durability is strictly limited to a partial day, at best. Taste buds and peripheral vision have disappeared along with my healthy immune system. Gone also is that happy-go-lucky exuberance of loving life, having a career and being fueled with the pleasant wonder and level of excitement the natural ease of contentment shrouded me in for so many years.

Survival is so much more than healing. It is the undaunting task of adaptability and conformity. Making the most of yourself after getting as well as you're going to get, allowing each breath to coincide with hope. My hope is that each day will be slightly better than the previous one, because I am still surviving, adapting and coping. Knowing that I can only make the best of what's left of me and the remainder of my human character. Each night I say goodbye to my way of life before the aneurysm. Each morning I say hello to the rest of my life.

The end

PROCLAMATION

WHEREAS, cerebrovascular death affects persons of all ages, sex, income and geographic locations; and

WHEREAS, an estimated 157,689 deaths in the United States occur each year from cerebrovascular incidents; and

WHEREAS, an average of 3,965 Tennesseeans die each year from cerebrovascular incidents; and

WHEREAS, an estimated 30,000 Americans suffer a cerebrovascular event known as a ruptured brain aneurysm (subarachnoid hemorrhage) each year; and

WHEREAS, 60% of these die before reaching the hospital, within 24 hours or within 30 days of the episode; and

WHEREAS, only 20% will be alive one year after the ruptured aneurysm; and

WHEREAS, 10 to 25% of these will have serious permanent damage caused by the death of nerve cells, and undergo long term rehab or nursing home admissions; and

WHEREAS, over half of the remaining survivors will have permanent neurological deficits including memory, speech and mobility impairments; and

WHEREAS, there is no known method to prevent a cerebral aneurysm.

NOW, THEREFORE, I, Phil Bredesen, Governor of the State of Tennessee, do hereby proclaim the day of January 25, 2007 as

BRAIN ANEURYSM SURVIVOR DAY

in Tennessee and encourage all citizens to join me in this worthy observance.

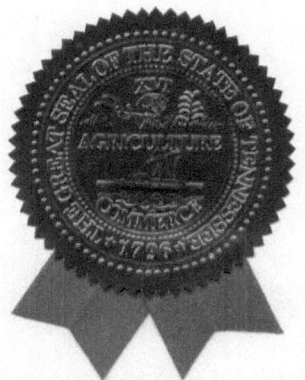

IN WITNESS WHEREOF, I have hereunto set my hand and caused the official seal of the State of Tennessee to be affixed at Nashville on this 4th day of October, 2006.

Governor

Secretary of State